Paediatric Pain Management
a multi-disciplinary approach

D1323308

Edited by

Alison Twycross
Anthony Moriarty
and Tracy Betts

Forewords by

Neil Morton
and Sue Price

RADCLIFFE MEDICAL PRESS

© 1998 Alison Twycross, Anthony Moriarty and Tracy Betts

Radcliffe Medical Press Ltd
18 Marcham Road, Abingdon, Oxon OX14 1AA, UK

British Library Cataloguing in Publication Data

A catalogue record for this book is available from the British Library.

ISBN 1 85775 246 5

Library of Congress Cataloging-in-Publication Data is available.

Typeset by Advance Typesetting Ltd, Oxon
Printed by TJI Digital, Padstow, Cornwall

Contents

Foreword

Pain in children has been under-diagnosed and under-treated for years. Recently, it has been realized that with good education, most paediatric pain can be safely and effectively prevented and controlled with existing techniques adapted for the age, maturity and severity of illness of the child. This requires attention to developmental, emotional and physical components when assessing, diagnosing and managing pain.

Integrating the special diagnostic and therapeutic knowledge and skills of many disciplines is vitally important in order that a uniform high standard of pain prevention and pain control can be achieved for all paediatric patients. This book brings these threads together in a clear and provocative way, drawing heavily on the large evidence base now available in the medical, nursing and psychology literature.

Those who read this book will have a better understanding of the available evidence in their particular field but will also appreciate what other disciplines have to offer. I hope this will inspire them to improve the prevention and control of pain in their own clinical area and to make contact with other disciplines to organize and integrate the service they provide to *all* children not just the lucky few.

Neil Morton
Consultant in Paediatric Anaesthesia
September 1997

Foreword

Research published during the 1970s and 1980s presented a gloomy picture of children's pain being ignored or under-treated. Researchers demonstrated that the assessment and management of the pain that children were experiencing was one of the most neglected aspects of the care of children and their families. There appeared to be little guidance for those who cared for children, with information about children's pain confined to just a few pages in textbooks.

Fortunately the 1990s have seen a change of attitude among health care professionals. It is now recognized that pain may be a feature of a significant number of children's lives during episodes of acute and chronic illness, in both hospital and community settings. It is considered increasingly important to foster the partnerships that are required between health care professionals to ensure that appropriate management of children's pain can be achieved. In this way both our knowledge and practice will develop for the ultimate benefit of children and their families.

Continuing improvement in the care of children in pain cannot be maintained without easy access to understandable information on the developments in this area of care. Such information should demonstrate the link between a clear theoretical understanding and effective practice based on sound research. In this way health care professionals can be encouraged to use effective assessment tools as a first step in the use of increasingly effective methods of managing children's pain.

This book, with its multi-disciplinary approach, will make an important contribution to the continued improvement of the care of children and their families when they are experiencing episodes of pain.

Sue Price
English National Board for Nursing,
Midwifery and Health Visiting
September 1997

Preface

'By any reasonable code, freedom from pain should be a basic human right limited only by our knowledge to achieve it' (Leibeskind and Melzack 1988)

While much work has been undertaken in the last 10 to 15 years in the area of paediatric pain management, in 1996 Cummings *et al.* found that children are still enduring unnecessary pain. This book has been written for all health care professionals who care for children. There is a need for all members of the multi-disciplinary team to work together to manage paediatric pain properly and for this reason contributions to this book have been made by nurses, doctors and clinical psychologists. This is a multi-disciplinary book intended to help all members of the health care team work together to ensure that children no longer endure unnecessary pain. It provides the theoretical knowledge required to manage paediatric pain with the information presented in an accessible manner so that the reader is then able to apply what they have learnt in their clinical practice. As health care professionals we have a duty to provide quality care to children and their families; quality care means striving to relieve children's pain and making this objective a priority. It is not enough to pay lip service to pain management – we must implement into everyday practices the theoretical knowledge that is currently available. It is only when we do so that children will no longer suffer unnecessary pain. This book provides the reader with the theoretical knowledge to enable this to happen.

Alison Twycross
September 1997

List of contributors

Tracy Betts RGN RSCN DPSN
Clinical Services Manager (Nursing)
Birmingham Children's Hospital NHS Trust
Ladywood Middleway
Birmingham B16 8ET

Pamela Johnson RGN RSCN DPSN BSc (Nursing) ENB405 HSM (Cert) C&G730
Clinical Nurse Specialist
Birmingham Children's Hospital NHS Trust
Ladywood Middleway
Birmingham B16 8ET

Dr Andrew Liley MB ChB FRCA
Consultant Anaesthetist
Birmingham Children's Hospital NHS Trust
Ladywood Middleway
Birmingham B16 8ET

Annie Mercer BA(Hons) MA Clin Psychol, Dip Psychotherapy
Consultant Clinical Psychologist
Alderhey Children's Hospital
Eaton Road
Liverpool L12 2AP

Dr Anthony Moriarty MB BS FRCA
Consultant Anaesthetist
Birmingham Children's Hospital NHS Trust
Ladywood Middleway
Birmingham B16 8ET

Anthony Schwartz MA Clin Psychol, MSc Medical Psychology
Chartered Clinical Psychologist
Crown House
Beecroft Road
Cannock
Staffs WS11 1JP

Dr Andrew Tatman MB BS BSc MRCP FRCA
Consultant Anaesthetist
Birmingham Children's Hospital NHS Trust
Ladywood Middleway
Birmingham B16 8ET

Anne Taylor RGN RSCN BSc(Hons) ENB219 C&G730 PGCE
Lecturer Practitioner in Children's Nursing
Children's Ward Nuffield Orthopaedic Centre NHS Trust
Headington
Oxford OX3 7LD

Alison Twycross RGN RMN RSCN MSc DMS
Senior Lecturer in Paediatric Nursing
University of Central England
Faculty of Health and Community Care
Westbourne Road
Birmingham B15 3TN

Acknowledgements

The editors wish to acknowledge the help and advice given to them by Ruth Day, Fiona Dobson, Bob Moloney, Robert Twycross and colleagues at the University of Central England and at Birmingham Children's Hospital.

1 Perceptions about paediatric pain

Introduction

'Pain is whatever the experiencing person says it is, existing wherever they say it does.'[1]

'An unpleasant sensory and emotional experience with actual or potential tissue damage, or described in terms of such damage. Pain is always subjective. Each individual learns the application of the word through experiences related to injury in early life.'[2]

These two well-known definitions of pain illustrate that the experience of pain is both subjective and an individual phenomenon. It is, therefore, not surprising that health care professionals encounter difficulties in the assessment and management of pain. The perceptions of health care professionals about pain are also influenced by their personal beliefs, attitudes and values.[3] The situation is exacerbated by the continuing belief in the misconceptions about paediatric pain that persist despite compelling evidence which proves them to be myths.[4,5] This chapter will demonstrate that children's pain is not managed appropriately in practice and will then explore the evidence that demonstrates the mythological status of the misconceptions about paediatric pain. The factors that influence health care professionals in their assessment of pain will then be discussed and finally consideration will be given to changing practice.

How well is children's pain managed in practice?

Seventy-five per cent of children were in pain on the day of surgery, and 40% in severe pain. Only slightly fewer patients reported moderate to severe pain on the first post-operative day. Children were not receiving sufficient analgesics post-operatively.[6]

The Royal College of Surgeons and College of Anaesthetists' report on *Pain After Surgery* states that several studies have shown that weaker oral analgesics were relied upon more frequently in children and fewer and relatively smaller doses of opioids were given compared with those for adults.[7]

McIlvaine indicates that nursing staff will not give opioid analgesia on a fixed schedule if the analgesics are ordered on an 'as necessary' (p.r.n.) basis. He suggests that the child must demonstrate a need for the analgesia and then suffer through the period between the request and relief.[8]

Mather and Mackie felt that this situation was due to several factors:[6]

- medical prescriptions were often inadequate

- nurses interpreted the p.r.n. prescriptions as meaning 'as little as possible'

- nurses were reluctant to give opiate analgesics, substituting non-opiates soon after surgery.

Other studies also found that pain in children was not managed effectively:

- Eland and Anderson compared the post-operative pain management of 18 adults with 25 children. Twelve of the children received a total of 24 doses of analgesics (13 non-opiates and 11 opiates), whereas the remaining 13 children were not given any analgesics. In contrast the adults received 372 doses of opiate and 299 doses of non-opiate analgesics[9]

- Schechter et al. reviewed the charts of 90 children and 90 adults with identical diagnoses and found that, in general, adults received twice as many doses of opioids as the children per hospital day. The longer the hospital stay the greater became the difference between adults and children[10]

- Beyer et al. compared the administration of analgesics to 50 children and 50 adults who had undergone cardiac surgery. Six children were prescribed no post-operative analgesics; adults received 70% of the analgesics administered; children received 30%[11]

- Eland reported that 66% of hospitalized children (n = 2000) aged four to 10 years received no analgesics for the relief of pain[12]

- Cummings et al. found, in 1996, that many children were still enduring unacceptable levels of pain during hospitalization.[13]

Analysis of these findings indicates that children's pain is still not being managed effectively. This has serious implications – not only are children suffering unnecessary pain but unrelieved pain has many undesirable consequences. The consequences of unrelieved pain are shown in Box 1.1.

Box 1.1   Consequences of unrelieved pain[14]

- Rapid shallow breathing that can lead to alkalosis

- Inadequate expansion of lungs that can lead to bronchiectasis and atelectasis

- Inadequate cough that can lead to retention of secretions

- Increased heart rate and tissue ischaemia; the patient will not move spontaneously and will not ambulate

- Fluid and electrolyte losses are increased resulting in rapid respiration and increased perspiration and an increased metabolic rate

- Psychological consequences resulting in nightmares about pain and surgery – the patient will be less co-operative in the future and will have increased anxiety

---

Initially, at least part of the problem with the management of children's pain was an inadequate research base. Research on paediatric pain, however, has proliferated in the last 15 years but health care professionals are still not managing pain appropriately.[15–17] It is difficult to establish exactly why this should be. It would appear to be partly a problem of implementing evidence-based practice. Significant contributions to the problem are the attitudes and beliefs about children in pain that are held by many health care professionals. These erroneous attitudes will now be discussed.

Misconceptions about paediatric pain

Nurses continue to have misconceptions about paediatric pain in spite of the compelling evidence that demonstrates that they are myths.[4,5]

It is clear that children's pain is not being managed adequately and a primary reason for this lies in the perceptions of the nurse caring for the child. A number of misconceptions about paediatric pain have been identified. Comprehensive summaries of these are provided by Burr,[18] Eland[12] and Hawley.[19] A list of these misconceptions can be seen in Box 1.2. These misconceptions have all been shown to have no scientific basis.[20,21]

Box 1.2   Misconceptions about paediatric pain

- Infants cannot feel pain because of immature nervous system
- Children do not feel as much pain as adults
- Active children are not in pain
- Sleeping children cannot be in pain
- Children always tell the truth about pain
- Injections are not painful
- Children cannot describe and/or locate their pain
- The child is crying because he or she is restrained not because he or she is in pain
- Parents know all the answers about children's pain
- Opiates are not safe for use with children

Infants *can* feel pain

It is clear that infants do feel pain; it could be considered that because infants are unable to make sense of the noxious stimuli they may feel more pain than an older child.

After considering the evidence below one is forced to agree with Owens that: 'The burden of proof should be shifted to those who maintain that infants do not feel pain.'[22]

- The belief that the infant is incapable of pain sensation and perception has been maintained by misunderstandings regarding the pain transmission mechanism, misconceptions about the infant's response capabilities and uncertainty about the infant's memory of pain.[23]
- Volpe has shown that complete myelination of the nervous system is not necessary for pain to be felt.[24]
- Nociceptive pathways to the central nervous system are not completely myelinated until the 30th week of gestation. Incomplete myelination,

however, implies only a slower conduction speed in the nerves, which is offset by the shorter distances the impulses have to travel.[25]

- McGrath describes nociception as the detection of a noxious stimulus and the transaction and transmission of information about the presence and quality of that stimulus from the site of stimulation to the brain. Nociception does not, therefore, involve evaluating or attributing meaning to the subjective experience called pain so it is possible for infants to feel pain even though they may not be able to make sense of the stimuli.[26]

- Even extremely pre-term infants can localize and withdraw from noxious stimuli. Crying and altered facial responses strongly suggest that they feel pain and experience distress.[27]

- Neonates in Franck's study all demonstrated a response to painful stimuli that consisted of immediate withdrawal of both legs followed by crying. The crying was often accompanied by vigorous gross motor activity involving facial grimacing and movement of all extremities.[28]

- Haslam found that tolerance to pain increases with age.[29]

Children *do* feel as much pain as adults

Children and adults behave differently when in pain but this does not mean that children experience less pain than adults.

- Children do feel pain and if a child and an adult break a leg, the message about the pain is the same. However, the way in which the adult and child behave in response to that broken leg may be entirely different.[12]

- 'To some extent children may be able to use certain coping strategies, such as distraction and physical activity, better than adults. Thus at times the child may be better able to tolerate pain than the adult, but the adult's overall ability to cope with pain is considerably greater than the child's. The adult with pain usually has more control over his situation, including more knowledge about pain relief measures… and more ability to persist in obtaining pain relief such as asking the doctor to increase a dose or request a consultation.'[30]

- There is nothing to suggest that pain in children, although different, is less severe than that experienced by adults.[7]

- Tolerance to pain actually increases with age.[29]

- Although the literature does not show conclusively that children experience the same pain as adults, there is also little evidence to support the assumption that children feel less pain than adults.[11]

An active or sleeping child *may be* in pain

When assessing a child's pain it is important to remember that just because the child is not lying on his or her bed, is active or is playing, this does not mean that he or she is not in pain.

- Pain may result in exhausted sleep; thus a sleeping child could be in pain.[19]
- Children read or watch television in order to distract themselves from the pain.[6]
- Children who remain in their beds can easily be found. If they can be found they can be examined, poked and prodded, or taken off to who knows where![31] It therefore makes sense to children to be active and to play in order to avoid painful experiences.
- Increased activity is often a sign of pain and is the way children cope with the pain they are experiencing. Children may not realize that resting a painful limb will decrease the amount of pain they are experiencing.[32]
- Children can use play as a diversion and coping mechanism;[1] children are particularly gifted in the use of distraction.[30]

Children *do not* always tell the truth about pain

Children may lie about their pain for a number of reasons.

- Fear of injections is a common reason for children to deny pain.[1,6,12,33]
- Children at any age may deny pain if the questioner is a stranger, if they believe they are supposed to be brave, if they are fearful, if they anticipate receiving an injection for pain, or to avoid any number of suspected harmful or undesirable events.[31,33,34]

- Nurses need to examine closely the reasons for a child's denial of pain and refusal of medication, as denial does not mean they are pain-free:
  - they may be scared of having an injection
  - not realize that analgesics can be given for pain in sites other than the operation site
  - think that the nurse realizes they are in pain.[19]

- Fear of addiction to opioids is prevalent among parents, adolescents and school-aged children; this may lead to denial of pain.[3,4]

- They may hope that by denying pain they will be discharged sooner and avoid painful treatments.

- Children under seven years of age may feel that the pain is a punishment for doing wrong and they may suffer in silence because they feel they deserve to be punished.[31,33]

> Health care professionals need to remember that children do not always tell the truth about pain and should use other methods of pain assessment such as non-verbal indicators.

Nowadays it is not necessary to administer analgesia via intra-muscular injections; children and their parents, however, continue to perceive injections as the only way of receiving analgesia. It is also important to remember that some children in pain may think they are being honest when telling you that they are not in pain – the onset of the pain is so gradual that they do not realize they have pain until it has been alleviated, resulting in what appears to be a deliberate denial of pain.

The best way to administer analgesics is *not* by intra-muscular injection. Injections *are* painful

> Children do not like injections. Nurses should endeavour to provide analgesia via alternative routes, e.g. orally, continuous infusions, intra-venous patient controlled analgesia and the use of pre-sited subcutaneous cannulae. Many children's hospitals are now virtually 'intra-muscular injection free zones'.
>
> An injection is probably the worst possible way to administer any drug to a child.[31]

- Sixty-two per cent of hospitalized children aged four to 10 years say that an injection is the 'worst hurt they've ever had'.[35]

- Children fear injections more than anything else in hospital.[6]

- If an adult was hit with a baseball bat when they admitted to having pain they would soon stop admitting to experiencing pain; to a child the injection is the baseball bat.[14]

- Children with cancer state that the worst type of pain is from 'shots'; bone-marrow aspirations and lumbar punctures do not occur very often, but 'shots' are a daily reality.[31]

In spite of what is known about the safety and effectiveness of other ways of administering opioid analgesics, intra-muscular drugs are still widely used to administer opiate analgesia with paediatric patients.

Adults know that the momentary pain of an injection is worth the benefit obtained. Children do not associate subsequent relief from an injection with the injection itself. Two events are only related in the eyes of a young child if they occur at the same time.[35]

Children *can* describe and locate their pain

If appropriate methods, such as pain assessment tools, are used children can communicate about their pain but they use fewer, and different, words to describe their pain.[36]

Nurses need to use the appropriate pain assessment tools, so that children are able to describe and locate their pain.

- It is unlikely that children will ever articulate their pain experiences as accurately as adults. They can and do, however, relate their pain and discomfort adequately using words such as hurt and sore.[31]

- McGrath reports that children as young as 18 months are able to report their pain verbally and localize it.[37]

- Children as young as three years have used self-report tools and can locate their pain.[9,38]

- Children can demonstrate on an outline of the body where they hurt, without knowing the names of the body parts.[32]

Children cry because they are in pain, *not* because they are being restrained

When health care professionals perform procedures on children and have to hold the child down to do so, they often try to convince themselves that they are not hurting the child. This is *not*, however, the case.

Health care professionals need to evaluate their practice in this area.

This is a coping mechanism used by nurses and doctors but this rationale should not be used to deny pain relief to any child. Procedures are easier to perform on co-operative children. It is more appropriate to use chemical restraints, such as analgesics, rather than physical restraint.[31]

Parents do *not* always know all the answers about their child's pain

While parents are the best source of information about their child they may never have seen their child in a pain-producing situation or be so stressed that they cannot focus on the pain.[12]

It is often assumed that parents know all the answers about their child's pain;[12] parents are expected to know when their child is in pain and nurses expect the parents to ask for pain relief for their child. Eland found that a parent's most frequent responses regarding pain were 'the nurse would know if my child was in pain and would take care of it', 'the nurse wouldn't let my child suffer' or 'I've never seen a child with this, but the nurse has taken care of many children with it and would know if my child hurt'.[31]

Parents are a great source of comfort to the child in hospital, serve as excellent distracters from things that hurt, and are great anxiety reducers.[33] The nurse needs to help parents identify ways in which they can help their child cope with the pain.

Opiates *are* safe for use in children

The use of opioids as analgesics is extremely unlikely to cause addiction in children.

'Fear of creating opioid addiction should never be a reason for withholding opioid analgesics from anyone who needs them for pain relief.'[33]

Many nurses and physicians believe that the risk of a patient becoming addicted to opioid analgesics is high and use this as a reason for their reluctance to administer them.[14] This appears to be due to a lack of understanding of addiction; McCaffery *et al.* found that less than 25% of nurses correctly identified the incidence of psychological dependence (addiction) to opioid analgesics.[39]

Addiction is defined as a psychological dependence – using the drug for psychological effects, not for medical reasons. Addiction occurs when people have a continued craving for an opiate and the need to use the drug for reasons other than pain.

• Morrison, in a study of children with sickle-cell crisis (n = 198), observed that in 423 episodes treated with continuous infusions of intravenous opioids only one child demonstrated addictive behaviour. This child's addiction could not be directly related to the use of opioids in the management of pain.[40]

• Dilworth and MacKellar administered over 600 continuous intravenous infusions of opioid analgesics; there were no cases of addiction.[41]

• Opiates are no more dangerous for children than adults; only four out of 11 882 hospitalized patients became addicted to narcotics and all four had a history of drug abuse.[42]

Physical dependence (withdrawal symptoms) is *not* the same as addiction.

• Physical dependence may occur within one week of using opioids.

• Withdrawal symptoms will not occur unless the opioid is withdrawn suddenly or an antagonist (such as naloxone) is given.

• Withdrawal symptoms will not occur if the opioid is gradually decreased.

- Withdrawal symptoms are rarely a problem in clinical practice and represent what happens when the body has become used to certain chemicals.[14,33]

Tolerance (the need for increased doses of opioids to produce effective analgesia) is *not* the same as addiction.

- Tolerance to both the analgesic effect and toxicity of opioids occurs with sustained use.[43]

- As tolerance develops, increasing doses of opioids are required to produce effective analgesia.[44]

Provided the dose is appropriate the risk of respiratory depression due to opioid analgesic use in children is minimal.

Although respiratory depression is a well-known side effect of opioid analgesics, health care professionals appear to have an exaggerated fear about the likelihood of it occurring and their ability to treat or control it.[3]

- The risk of respiratory depression in children is no greater than in adults provided the dose is appropriate.[12,41,45]

- Minor respiratory depression occurred in 5% of the children but it had not been the source of anxiety that nurses and physicians feared; it had been promptly recognized and easily corrected.[41]

- The reluctance of health care professionals to use opiates in children is due to their inexperience in administering them to this age group.[12]

- The risk of using opiates in children is no greater than using them in adults.[30,46]

In the face of the evidence discussed, it is hard to understand how misconceptions about paediatric pain can still exist. The continuing existence of the belief in the misconceptions by health care professionals results in children continuing to feel unnecessary pain during hospitalization.

A summary of the misconceptions and evidence can be seen in Box 1.3.

Box 1.3 Misconceptions and evidence

Misconceptions	Facts
Infants cannot feel pain because of immature nervous system	Complete myelination not necessary for pain to be felt[24]
	Neonates exhibit behavioural, physiological and hormonal responses to pain[22,25,28,]
Children do not feel as much pain as adults	Tolerance to pain increases with age[29]
Opiates cause respiratory depression and addiction	The risk of respiratory depression is no greater than in adults provided the dose is appropriate[45]
	Opiates are no more dangerous for children than adults[42]
	No incidences of addiction in post-operative children shown[41]
	Fear of creating opioid addiction should never be a reason for withholding opioid analgesics from anyone who needs them for pain relief[33]
Active children are not in pain	Increased activity is often a sign of pain[12]
A child engaged in playing activities cannot be in pain	Children can use play as a diversion and coping mechanism[1]
	Children are particularly gifted in the use of distraction[31]
Sleeping children cannot be in pain	Pain may result in exhausted sleep[19]
Children always tell the truth about pain	Children may not admit to pain because of fear of the 'needle' or being ignored[1,12]
	Fear of what will happen next may prevent them from disclosing the truth[6]
Injections are not painful	62% of hospitalized children aged four to ten years say that an injection is the 'worst hurt they've ever had'[35]
	Children fear injections more than anything else in hospital[6]

Box 1.3 Continued	
Misconceptions	Facts
Children cannot describe and/or locate their pain	Children as young as three years have used self-report tools and can locate their pain[9,39]
Parents know all the answers about children's pain	Parents are the best source of information about their child but may never have seen the child in a pain-producing situation or be so stressed that they cannot focus on the pain[12]
	Parents feel that the nurse would know if their child was in pain[12]

Nurses' perceptions of pain

Nurses document less than 50% of the pain their patients describe.[47]

Health care professionals' perceptions of children's pain are not always accurate.[48]

Nurses rely on intuitions, assumptions and personal beliefs in order to assess children's pain.[49]

A primary role of the nurse should be to relieve pain,[12] but the misconceptions discussed previously lead to problems with how nurses perceive paediatric pain. Nurses often do not perceive correctly the amount of pain a child is experiencing:

- nurses, in general, underestimated the amount of pain experienced by the children. This was particularly pronounced after analgesics had been administered; nurses tended to overestimate the effect of analgesics[50]

- pain assessment in children and subsequent decisions to medicate are inconsistent with what is known about the experience of pain in childhood[51]

- pain ratings made by the child, parent and nurse reflect different perspectives.[52]

Nurses underestimate the amount of pain their patients experience, relying on intuitions, assumptions and personal beliefs to assess pain. This results in children continuing to suffer unnecessary pain.

Pain relief is a low priority among nurses and other health care professionals.[53-55]

Five per cent of the respondents in a study reported by Gadish et al. said it was their aim to relieve pain completely, while 63% aimed to relieve pain as much as possible. Twenty-four per cent of the nurses aimed to relieve only enough pain for the patient to function.[51]

In 1995, 57% of nurses in a study reported by Caty et al. stated that the goal of giving medication was complete relief of pain; 24% said their goal was to keep pain at a tolerable level or to provide enough pain relief so that pain is noticed but is not distressing.[15]

Nurses tend to concentrate on the technical aspects of care rather than assessing children's pain,[5] indicating that relieving pain is not seen as a priority. No nurse likes to inflict pain, but relieving it has always received low priority.[56] The majority of nurses think that pain is related to hospital admission; some of them think pain can never be relieved completely – 'In fact, some pain is allowed, for they are, after all, in hospital'.[57] The low priority that nurses give to relieving pain compounds a situation where children are already suffering unnecessary pain.

Influences affecting nurses' perception of pain

Studies suggest that health care professionals are subject to various influences when assessing pain, including their own experiences of pain.[3,15]

A summary of factors which influence nurses' perceptions of pain in adults can be seen in Box 1.4.

Several studies have demonstrated that the majority of nurses thought that adults experience more pain than children in the same situation.[9-11]

Box 1.5 summarizes the studies that have identified factors that influence nurses' perceptions of pain in children.

Box 1.4   Factors that influence nurses' perceptions of pain in adults

- Personal pain histories[58]
- Length of nursing experience[59-63]
- Educational level[61]
- Membership of a professional group such as the oncology nurses forum[61]
- Nurses' knowledge about observable behaviours[64]
- Personal belief systems about meaning of observable phenomenon[64]
- Positive physical pathology[63]
- Gender[64]

Health care professionals need to be aware of these influencing factors, that could result in possible biases in their pain assessment and management.

Many of the factors that influence nurses' perceptions of pain in children are not well researched. There is a need for further research,[65] particularly in the area of culture and children's temperament.

A number of studies have found that nurses rely heavily on a child's vital signs as a primary tool for assessment purposes.[17,51,70] Physiological variables, however, do not reflect perception of pain as the body adapts to stressors by homoeostasis, and so these variables may not be helpful in assessing pain.[71] It is no wonder that nurses continue to perceive children's pain inaccurately.

Inadequate education

Basic nurse education has the biggest influence on nursing practice with regard to pain management.[51]

The greatest hurdle to overcome in providing relief of pain to children remains the education of colleagues and parents.[8]

A major cause for undermedication of cancer pain is inadequate education among those who provide the care.[4]

Box 1.5   Factors that influence nurses' perceptions of pain in children

- *Having a child who has had a painful episode* – nurses are not influenced by their own pain experiences. If their own child has suffered a painful episode, however, this does appear to influence decisions regarding the administration of analgesics[53]

- *Type of unit in which the patient is nursed* – nurses in the paediatric intensive care unit used opioids more frequently than non-opioid analgesics[53]

- *Priority that nurses afford pain management* – if a nurse who assesses a child in pain sees pain relief as a priority the child will receive medication for its pain[53]

- *Educational background of nurse* – the greater the educational background, the higher the dose of opioid analgesics selected[51]

- *Age of child* – The pre-verbal child received the greatest amount of non-opiate and lower dosage opiate analgesia[51]

- *Time since surgery* – there was a reliance on the time elapsed since surgery as an indicator of pain intensity and need for analgesic administration[65]

- *Medical diagnosis* – the presence of a medical diagnosis appeared to justify being in pain and to justify partly the administration of analgesics[57,65]

- *Child's temperament/behaviour/expression* – a shouting or crying child will be administered an analgesic sooner than a child who does not react in a verbal manner [5,57,66]

- *Nurse's attitude* – nurses have negative feelings regarding analgesics and they postpone giving them for as long as possible [57]

- *Nurse's past experience of children in pain* – nurses use their past experiences to determine how to manage a child's pain[5,57]

- *Nurse's knowledge about effects of pain relieving interventions* – nurses with a greater knowledge regarding opiate analgesics appeared more comfortable with administering them and give higher doses[57,67]

- *Nurse's workload* – nurses often do not have time to implement pain relief methods for children[1,57]

- *Culture* – health care professionals are often ethnocentric;[68] culture or ethnicity is an important consideration with respect to children's pain, manifesting its influence through attitudes, such as 'the meaning' of illness and pain, and through learned behaviour patterns and norms[69]

Traditionally, little space has been allocated to pain management in the nursing curriculum.

- Of the 15 472 pages in the ten most frequently used paediatric textbooks, only 3.5 pages were found to be devoted to discussion of pain and related topics.[72]

- The teaching received in training did not appear to have left the sample nurses with knowledge of methods of pain assessment and control.[17]

- Nurse educators should pay more attention to pain assessment and to methods of relieving pain in children.[56]

- Some nurses were not aware of current paediatric pain knowledge and did not use these advancements in the assessment and management of paediatric pain.[15]

If perceptions about pain are to change, more time needs to be allocated to pain management in nursing and medical curricula. One or two post-registration courses on paediatric pain management are now run in Britain; there is a need for more. McCaffery reminds us that there is always a time lag between the identification of information and its dissemination to those who need it.[73] As well as improving the educational input regarding paediatric pain management, methods need to be found to facilitate evidence-based practice.

Doctors' perceptions

Nurses and physicians use similar words to describe pain.[74]

Nurses and doctors perceive pain in children in the same way; there is a lack of knowledge among nurses and doctors about the appropriate dosages of pain medication.[75]

There is very little information regarding doctors' perceptions of paediatric pain. It can be concluded from the studies cited above that the factors that influence nurses' perceptions of pain also influence doctors' perceptions. Mather and Mackie in their investigation into the amount of pain suffered by children post-operatively found that medical prescriptions were often inadequate.[6] It is, therefore, possible to assume that doctors do not perceive accurately the pain experienced by their patients. Research has shown that nurses continue to have misconceptions about paediatric pain;[4,5] anecdotal evidence demonstrates that this is the case for doctors as well. There is, therefore, a need for doctors to be aware of misconceptions about paediatric pain and of the factors that may influence their perceptions of a child's pain. This area appears to be under-researched.

Parents' perceptions

Only 17% of nurses used parents' assessments when assessing a child's pain, ranking it the lowest indicator of pain.[57]

Nurses do not usually rely on parental input when assessing the child's pain.[76]

Nurses and parents found it hard to work together to manage children's pain.[77]

Parents are well aware of their children's history of pain and their usual ways of coping with it; they can provide valuable baseline data for the nurse to use in decision making.[31] As previously stated, parents are the best source of information about their children but they may never have seen their children in a pain-producing situation or they may be so stressed that they cannot focus on the pain.[12]

Parents are a great source of comfort to the child in hospital, serve as excellent distracters from things that hurt, and are great anxiety reducers.[5,31]

Parents are a comfort to their child during painful experiences but are they able to rate their child's level of pain intensity? Watt-Watson et al. examined parents' perceptions of their child's acute pain experience and found that parents were able to identify the non-verbal clues which indicated that their child was in pain.[78] Parents in the study identified a lack of information about painful procedures, of prognoses related to pain duration, and of effective comfort measures for their child. There is, therefore, a need for nurses and doctors to provide better information for parents.

Miller found that mothers may be a valuable source of information regarding their child's pain and should be included in the assessment process.[79] Nurses need to educate mothers and fathers regarding the importance of their perceptions and encourage them to participate in assessing their child's pain. Parents are a valuable asset in the management of children's pain. Box 1.6 lists the implications for practice of the research into parents' perceptions of their child's pain. Further research is indicated in this area.

Box 1.6   Parents' perceptions of pain – implications for practice

---

- Parents are a valuable asset in the management of children's pain

- Parents are able to identify non-verbal clues which indicate that their child is in pain

- Parents require information about the pain and how it will be managed

- Parents need to be actively encouraged to participate in pain management

- Parents' ratings of pain intensity correlate closer with the child's than nurses' ratings

---

Health care professionals need to encourage parents to become involved in the pain assessment process; there is need for the provision of information and for parents to be actively encouraged to tell nurses when they think their child is in pain.

Changing attitudes and beliefs

'Many believe that when well-meaning people are educated about a phenomenon, their behaviour changes automatically. This is clearly not the case. A change of attitude or knowledge about pain management does not necessarily lead to changes in behaviour.'[80]

Burokas showed that personally held beliefs of nurses influence their decisions about medicating children after surgery.[53] Thus health care professionals need to examine their beliefs regarding pain and how these relate to their perceptions of effective pain management.[16] Even when attitudes change behaviour does not always alter. McGrath cites an example of an educational booklet for parents decreasing the negative attitudes towards medications in a sample of parents caring for a child post-operatively. There were, however, no changes in medication use or the pain experienced by the children.[80] Attitudes are relatively stable entities but are not fixed. They change and can be changed.[81] Changing beliefs and attitudes is never easy, which perhaps explains why, in spite of compelling evidence, health care professionals continue to have misconceptions. Zajonc[82] states that 'the mere repeated exposure of an individual to a stimulus has been shown to be sufficient to enhance his or her attitude to it.'

The challenge for all involved in paediatrics is how to change the behaviour of nurses, doctors and other heath care professionals in relation to pain management. The provision of information alone is not enough.

Summary

- Children are still enduring unnecessary pain.

- Misconceptions about paediatric pain are still prevalent in clinical practice today and these contribute to the unnecessary pain experienced by children.

- Nurses and doctors continue to have these misconceptions.

- A number of factors influence individual nurses and doctors when they assess a child's pain.

- A need for further education has been identified.

- Nurses must be the members of the health care team who assume accountability for pain control.[3]

- There is a need for children, parents, doctors, nurses and all members of the multi-disciplinary team to work in partnership to ensure that children no longer endure unnecessary pain.

> 'By any reasonable code, freedom from pain should be a basic human right limited only by our knowledge to achieve it.'[83]

References

1   McCaffery M (1972) *Nursing Management of the Patient with Pain.* Lippincott, Philadelphia.
2   International Association of the Study of Pain, Subcommittee on Taxonomy (1979) Pain terms: a list with definitions and notes on usage. *Pain.* **6**: 249–52.
3   Stevens B, Hunsberger M and Browne G (1987) Pain in children: theoretical, research and practice dilemmas. *Pediatr Nurs.* **2** (3): 154–66.
4   Schmidt K, Eland J and Weller K (1994) Pediatric cancer pain management: a survey of nurses' knowledge. *J Pediatr Oncol.* **11** (1): 4–12.
5   Woodgate R and Kristjanson LJ (1996) A young child's pain: how parents and nurses 'take care'. *Int J Nurs Stud.* **33** (3): 271–84.
6   Mather L and Mackie J (1983) The incidence of post-operative pain in children. *Pain.* **15**: 271–82.
7   The Royal College of Surgeons and College of Anaesthetists (1990) *Pain After Surgery.* RCS, London.

8   McIlvaine WB (1989) Perioperative pain management in children: a review. *J Pain Symptom Manage.* **4** (4): 215–29.

9   Eland JM and Anderson JE (1977) The experience of pain in children, In: *Pain: a sourcebook for nurses and other health care professionals* (ed. AK Jacox). Little, Brown & Company, Boston, pp. 453–73.

10 Schechter NL, Allen DA and Hanson K (1986) Status of paediatric pain control: a comparison of hospital analgesic usage in children and adults. *Pediatrics.* **77** (1): 11–15.

11 Beyer JE, DeGood DE, Ashley LC *et al.* (1983) Patterns of postoperative analgesic use with adults and children following cardiac surgery. *Pain.* **17**: 71–81.

12 Eland J (1985) Myths about pain in children. *The Candlelighters Childhood Cancer Foundation.* **V** (1), June.

13 Cummings EA, Reid GJ, Finley A *et al.* (1996) Prevalence and source of pain in pediatric inpatients. *Pain.* **68**: 25–31.

14 Eland J (1990) Pain in children. *Nurs Clin North Am.* **25** (4): 871–84.

15 Caty S, Tourigny J and Koren I (1995) Assessment and management of children's pain in community hospitals. *J Adv Nurs.* **22**: 638–45.

16 Margolius FR, Hudson KA and Michel Y (1995) Beliefs and perceptions about children in pain: a survey. *Pediatr Nurs.* **21** (2): 111–15.

17 Nethercott SG (1994) The assessment and management of post-operative pain in children by registered sick children's nurses: an exploratory study. *J Clin Nurs.* **3**: 109–14.

18 Burr S (1987) Pain in childhood. *Nursing.* **24**: 890–95.

19 Hawley D (1984) Postoperative pain in children: Misconceptions, descriptions and interventions. *Pediatr Nurs.* **10** (1): 20–3.

20 Ross DM and Ross SA (1984) The importance of type of question, psychological climate and subject set in interviewing children about pain. *Pain.* **19**: 71–9.

21 Bradshaw C and Zeanah PD (1986) Pediatric nurses' assessments of pain in children. *Pediatr Nurs.* **1** (5): 314–21.

22 Owens ME (1984) Pain in infancy: conceptual and methodological issues. *Pain.* **20**: 213–30.

23 Stevens BJ, Johnston CC and Grunau RVE (1995) Issues of assessment of pain and discomfort in neonates. *J Obstet Gynecol Neonatal Nurses.* **24** (9): 849–55.

24 Volpe J (1981) *Neurology of the Newborn.* Saunders, Philadelphia.

25 Anand KJS and Hickey PR (1987) Pain and its effects in the human neonate and fetus. *N Engl J Med.* **317** (21): 1321–9.

26 McGrath PA (1990) *Pain in Children: nature, assessment and treatment.* The Guildford Press, New York.

27 Porter F (1993) Pain assessment in children: infants. In: *Pain in Infants, Children and Adolescents* (eds NL Schechter, CB Berde and M Yaster). Williams & Wilkins, Baltimore, pp. 87–96.

28 Franck LS (1986) A new method to quantitatively describe pain behaviour in infants. *Nurs Res.* **35** (1): 28–31.

29 Haslam D (1969) Age and perception of pain. *Psychon Sci.* **15**: 86–7.

30 McCaffery M and Beebe AB (1989) *Pain: Clinical Manual for Nursing Practice.* CV Mosby, St Louis.

31 Eland J (1985) The child who is hurting. *Semin Oncol Nurs.* **1** (2): 116–22.

32   Eland J (1985) The role of the nurse in children's pain. In: *Recent Advances in Nursing: Perspectives on Pain* (ed. L Copp). Churchill Livingstone, Edinburgh.

33   McCaffery M and Wong DL (1993) Nursing interventions for pain control in children. In: *Pain in Infants, Children and Adolescents* (eds NL Schechter, CB Berde and M Yaster). Williams & Wilkins, Baltimore, pp. 295–316.

34   McGrath PJ, Unrah AM and Finlay GA (1995) Pain measurement in children. *Pain: Clinical Update.* **3** (2): 1–4.

35   Eland J (1981) Minimising pain associated with pre-kindergarten intra-muscular injections. *Issues Comprehensive Pediatr Nurs.* **5**: 361–72.

36   Wilkie DJ, Holzemer WL, Tesler MD *et al.* (1990) Measuring pain quality: validity and reliability of children's and adolescents' pain language. *Pain.* **41**: 151–9.

37   McGrath PA (1989) Evaluating a child's pain. *J Pain Symptom Manage.* **4**: 198–214.

38   Beyer JE and Wells N (1989) The assessment of pain in children. *Pediatr Clin North Am.* **36** (4): 837–54.

39   McCaffery M, Ferrell B, O'Neil-Page E *et al.* (1990) Nurses' knowledge of opioid analgesic drugs and psychological dependence. *Cancer Nurs.* **13** (1): 21–7.

40   Morrison RA (1991) Update on sickle cell disease: incidence of addiction and choice of opioid in pain management. *Pediatr Nurs.* **17** (5): 503.

41   Dilworth NM and MacKellar A (1987) Pain relief for the pediatric surgical patient. *J Pediatr Surg.* **22** (3): 264–8.

42   Porter J and Jick H (1980) Addiction rare in patients treated with narcotics. *N Engl J Med.* **302** (2): 123.

43   Miser AW (1993) Management of pain associated with childhood cancer. In: *Pain in Infants, Children and Adolescents* (eds NL Schechter, CB Berde and M Yaster). Williams & Wilkins, Baltimore, pp. 411–23.

44   Yaster M and Maxwell LG (1993) Opioid agonists and antagonists. In: *Pain in Infants, Children and Adolescents* (eds NL Schechter, CB Berde and M Yaster). Williams & Wilkins, Baltimore, pp. 145–71.

45   Miller RR and Jick H (1978) Clinical effects of meperidine in hospitalized medical patients. *J Clin Pharmacol.* **April**: 180–9.

46   American Pain Society (APS) (1989) *Principles of Analgesic Use in the Treatment of Acute Pain and Chronic Cancer Pain: A Concise Guide to Medical Practice.* (2nd edn) Skokie, Illinois.

47   Camp LD and O'Sullivan PS (1987) Comparison of medical, surgical and oncology patient's descriptions of pain and nurses' documentation of pain assessments. *J Adv Nurs.* **12**: 593–8.

48   Ellis JA (1988) Using pain scales to prevent undermedication. *MCN.* **13**: 180–2.

49   Beyer JE and Byers M (1985) Knowledge of pediatric pain. *Child Health Care.* **13** (4): 150–9.

50   Romsing J, Moller-Sonnergaard J, Hertel S *et al.* (1996) Postoperative pain in children: comparison between ratings of children and nurses. *J Pain Symptom Manage.* **11** (1): 42–6.

51   Gadish HS, Gonzalez JL and Hayes JS (1988) Factors affecting nurses' decisions to administer pediatric pain medication post-operatively. *Pediatr Nurs.* **3** (6): 383–9.

52   Manne SL, Jacobsen PB and Redd WH (1992) Assessment of acute paediatric pain: Do child self-report, parent ratings, and nurse ratings measure the same phenomenon? *Pain.* **48**: 45–52.

53   Burokas L (1985) Factors affecting nurses' decisions to medicate pediatric patients after surgery. *Heart Lung.* **14** (4): 373–8.

54   Abu-Saad H (1984) Assessing children's response to pain. *Pain.* **19**: 163–71.

55   Cohen FL (1980) Postsurgical pain relief: Patient's status and nurses' medication choices. *Pain.* **9**: 265–74.

56   McGuire L (1983) 7 myths about pain relief. *RN.* December 30: 33.

57   Hamers JPH, Abu-Saad HH, Halfens RJG and Schumacher JNM (1994) Factors influencing nurses' pain assessment and interventions in children. *J Adv Nurs.* **20**: 853–60.

58   Holm K, Cohen F, Dudas S *et al.* (1989) Effect of personal pain experience on pain assessment. *Image J Nurs Sch.* **21** (2): 72–5.

59   Davitz JR and Davitz LL (1981) *Influences on Patient's Pain and Distress.* Springer-Verlag, New York.

60   Mason DJ (1981) An investigation of the influences of selected factors on nurses' inferences of patient suffering. *Int J Nurs Stud.* **18** (4): 251–9.

61   Dalton JA (1989) Nurses' perceptions of their pain assessment skills, pain management practices, and attitudes towards pain. *Oncol Nurs Forum.* **16** (2): 225–31.

62   Dudley SR and Holm K (1984) Assessment of the pain experience in relation to selected nurse characteristics. *Pain.* **18**: 179–86.

63   Halfens R, Evers G and Abu-Saad H (1990) Determinants of pain assessment by nurses. *Int J Nurs Stud.* **27** (1): 43–9.

64   McCaffery M and Ferrell BR (1992) Does the gender gap affect your pain control? *Nursing.* **August**: 48–51.

65   Bush RS, Bush JP and Crummette BD (1991) Factors affecting nurses' decisions to administer PRN analgesic medication to children after surgery: an analog investigation. *J Ped Psychol.* **16** (2): 151–67.

66   Wallace MR (1989) Temperament: a variable in children's pain management. *Pediatr Nurs.* **15** (2): 118–21.

67   McGuire L and Dizard S (1982) Managing pain in the young patient. *Nursing.* **12**: 52, 54–5.

68   Martinelli AM (1987) Pain and ethnicity: how people of different cultures experience pain. *AORN J.* **46** (2): 273–4, 276, 278, 280–1.

69   Bernstein BA and Pachter LM (1993) Cultural considerations in children's pain. In: *Pain in Infants, Children and Adolescents* (eds NL Schechter, CB Berde and M Yaster). Williams & Wilkins, Baltimore, pp. 113–22.

70   Price PS (1992) Student nurses' assessment of children in pain. *J Adv Nurs.* **17**: 441–7.

71   Gildea JH and Quirk TR (1977) Assessing the pain experience in children. *Nurs Clin North Am.* **1**: 631–7.

72   Rana SR (1987) Pain – a subject ignored. *Pediatrics.* **79**: 309.

73   McCaffery M (1994) Commentary – pediatric cancer pain management: a survey of nurses' knowledge. *J Pediatr Oncol Nurs.* **11** (1): 13.

74   Norvell KT, Gaston-Johansson F and Zimmerman L (1990) Pain descriptions by nurses and physicians. *J Pain Symptom Manage.* **5** (1): 11–17.

75   Read JV (1994) Perceptions of nurses and physicians regarding pain management of pediatric emergency room patients. *Pediatr Nurs.* **20** (3): 314–18.

76   O'Brien SW and Konsler GK (1988) Alleviating children's postoperative pain. *MCN.* **13**: 183–6.

77 Woodgate R and Kristjanson LJ (1996) 'Getting better from my hurts': toward a model of the young child's pain experience. *Pediatr Nurs.* **11** (4): 233–42.
78 Watt-Watson JH, Everndern C and Lawson C (1990) Parents' perceptions of their child's acute pain experience. *Pediatr Nurs.* **5** (5): 344–9.
79 Miller D (1996) Comparisons of pain ratings from postoperative children, their mothers, and their nurses. *Pediatr Nurs.* **22** (2): 45–9.
80 McGrath PJ (1996) Attitudes and beliefs about medication and pain management in children. *J Palliat Care.* **12** (3): 46–50.
81 Downie RS, Fyfe C and Tannahill A (1990) *Health Promotion: Models and Values.* Oxford University Press, Oxford.
82 Zajonc RB (1968) In: *Health Promotion: Models and Values* (eds RS Downie, C Fyfe and A Tannahill). Oxford University Press, Oxford, p. 111.
83 Leibeskind JC and Melzack R (1988) The International Pain Foundation: meeting a need for education in pain management. *J Pain Symptom Manage.* **3** (3): 131–2.

Further reading

Broome ME and Slack JF (1990) Influences on nurses' management of pain in children. *MCN.* **15**: 158–62.

Favaloro R and Touzel B (1990) A comparison of adolescents' and nurses' postoperative pain ratings and perceptions. *Pediatr Nurs.* **16** (4): 414–24.

Ferrell BR, McCaffery M and Rhiner M (1992) Pain and addiction: an urgent need for change in nursing education. *J Pain Symptom Manage.* **7** (2): 117–24.

Grossman S, Sheidler VR, Swedeen K *et al.* (1991) Correlations of patient and caregiver ratings of cancer pain. *J Pain Symptom Manage.* **6** (2): 53–7.

Pigeon H, McGrath PJ, Lawrence J *et al.* (1989) Nurses' perceptions of pain in the neonatal intensive care unit. *J Pain Symptom Manage.* **4** (4): 179–83.

Teske K, Daut RL and Cleeland CS (1983) Relationships between nurses' observations and patients' self-reports of pain. *Pain.* **16**: 289–96.

Walsh M and Ford P (1989) It can't hurt that much! *Nurs Times.* **85** (42): 35–8.

2 Children's cognitive level and their perception of pain

How children perceive the cause and effect of pain changes as they mature; a five year-old child describes a painful event in a different manner to a 13 year-old. The reasons why nurses should seek to understand how children conceptualize illness and view the cause and effect of pain will be discussed in this chapter. Implications for nursing practice and pain management will also be identified.

Why nurses need to understand how children conceptualize illness

'An appreciation of the child's conception of illness can foster empathy, facilitate explanations of illness and medical procedures, and improve health education.'[1]

An understanding of how children develop a concept of illness will enhance the quality of care that nurses, and other health care professionals, provide. It has been shown that most doctors and nurses do not approach children according to their developmental levels but, rather, address all children as if they were in Piaget's concrete operational stage.[2] Knowledge about how a child's understanding of illness develops will mean that age-appropriate explanations can be given to children, thus reducing the anxiety and psychological distress children suffer during hospitalization.

'Optimal communication between providers of child health care and their patients depends on appropriate expectations of what the children can understand.'[2]

If nurses have knowledge about a child's level of understanding they will be able to:[3]

- help improve explanations of illness and hospitalization

- provide sensitive reassurance for children

- gain greater understanding of what the child is saying to them

- gain some insight into how the child is interpreting all the strange occur-
  rences that can accompany illness.

Development of understanding about the cause and effect of illness

Children develop a concept of illness which parallels Piaget's stages of cognitive development.[4-7]

Piaget's pre-operational stage

'During the pre-operational period, children are not able to distance
themselves from their environment. Their explanations for illness consist
of a simple cause and effect relationship, based on the specific spatial
and temporal cues in children's environments.'[8]

Pre-logical thinking is typical of children aged two to seven years. Children
are unable to distance themselves from their environment. There are two
types of pre-logical explanations for illness: *phenomenism* and *contagion*.
Phenomenism is the most developmentally immature explanation of illness.
The cause of illness is perceived as an external concrete phenomenon that
occurs at the same time as the illness but is spatially or temporally remote.
For example, when asked how people get colds, a child at this stage might
answer 'From the sun.' The explanatory stage called contagion is offered by
the more mature pre-operational child. The cause of illness is located in
objects or people that are close to, but not touching, the child. The link
between the cause and illness is accounted for only in terms of proximity
or by magical acts. A child at this stage would, for example, think that 'you
got a cold because you are near someone who has a cold.' A child of this
age would also think that more serious illnesses, such as leukaemia, were
'caught' by being in close proximity to someone suffering from a particular
illness.

Piaget's concrete operational stage

'The major developmental shift into the concrete operational period occurs when children begin to differentiate between themselves and others. Children begin to distinguish their internal from their external states to distinguish between the cause of illness and its effects. The cause is viewed as a person, object, or action that is external to the child and that has an aspect or quality that is bad or harmful to the body.'[8]

Children aged seven to 10 years exhibit concrete-logical thinking. The major developmental shift, according to Piaget, is the differentiation between self and other. The child begins to distinguish internal from external. The two illness explanations characteristic of this group are *contamination* and *internalization*.

Contamination is used most frequently by the younger children within this age group. The child perceives the cause of illness as a person, object or action external to the child that is 'bad' or 'harmful' to the body. For example, 'getting a cold because you didn't wear a coat' or 'getting pneumonia because you swam in the cold sea'. The perceived cause effects illness through physical contact or through the child engaging in harmful action and becoming contaminated.

Internalization, the second level of concrete-logical explanations, explains illness as located within the body although its ultimate cause remains external. An example of this thinking is 'getting a cold by breathing in air and bacteria' or 'getting leukaemia by breathing in bacteria'. The illness is now located within the body but is still described in vague terms. Confusion regarding internal organs and functions is still evident.

Piaget's formal operational stage

'During the formal operational stage children begin to think about and understand the world in more abstract terms. They may attribute illness to physiological or psychological causes.'[8]

Children of 11 years and older manifest formal-logical thinking. There is a greater amount of differentiation between self and others at this stage than during the previous stages. Children at this stage use *physiological* and *psychophysiological* explanations regarding illness.

Physiological explanations describe the cause of illness as a malfunctioning or non-functioning organ or process. Even though the cause may be triggered by external events, the source and nature of the illness is in a specific internal physiological structure or function. Children at this stage are able to explain their illness as a sequence of events. Psychophysiological explanations represent the most mature understanding of illness. The child realizes that psychological attitudes affect health and illness. The illness is described in terms of internal physiological processes, with consideration given to the psychological factors involved. For example, a heart attack is seen as a heart malfunctioning, which is brought about by tension and stress. However, personal clinical experience suggests that not all children (or even adults) reach this stage. A summary of how children perceive the cause and effect of illness can be seen in Box 2.1.

> Children's understanding of disease and treatment is determined more by age than by gender, socio-economic status or maternal understanding of the disease.[9]

Recently there has been a shift away from the traditional Piagetian emphasis on the child moving through a series of stages towards the view that what really changes is the content of knowledge.[10] However, it is knowledge that determines a child's level of understanding. The fact that the health care professionals do not take children's level of understanding, or stage of cognitive development, into account will affect the quality of the care they receive. Further research in this area is needed.

Development of understanding about the cause and effect of pain

> 'A child's cognitive level may have a significant effect on their perception and report of pain. Lack of communicative ability may prevent a child from adequately expressing the pain they are feeling. Also a lack of knowledge of the hospital environment may inhibit the child from asking for pain relief ... Pain is an abstract concept and for the young child in the early stages of cognitive development, the term pain may be meaningless.'[1]
>
> 'Since effective alleviation of children's pain requires an understanding of how they perceive pain, it is important to evaluate their developmental level to provide an appropriate course of therapy or pain management.'[8]

Box 2.1   How children perceive the cause and effect of illness[4,5,7]

Piaget's stage of development	Perception of illness
Pre-operational (2–7 years)	*Phenomenism* Cause of illness perceived as an external concrete phenomenon which occurs at the same time as the illness
	Contagion Cause of illness located in objects or people that are close to, but not touching the child
	Link between cause and illness due to proximity or magic
Concrete operational (7–11 years)	*Contamination* Cause of illness is a person, object or action external to the child that is 'bad' or 'harmful' to the body
	Perceived cause affects illness through physical contact or child engaging in harmful activity
	Internalization Illness is located within the body although its ultimate cause remains external
	Still described in vague terms
Formal operational (12 years and above)	*Physiological* Cause of illness described as a malfunctioning or non-functioning organ or process
	Able to describe their illness in a sequence of events
	Psychophysiological Realizes that psychological actions and attitudes affect health and illness
	Illness described in terms of internal physiological processes with consideration given to psychological factors

Pain threshold increases with age;[11] the younger a child the lower his or her pain threshold will be. Just because children cannot tell the nurse that they are in pain does not mean that they are not experiencing pain. Young children demonstrate behavioural clues that demonstrate that they are experiencing pain. The non-verbal clues which children use should always be considered when assessing pain. In order to assess children's pain, therefore, a nurse needs to have an understanding of how children of different ages and developmental levels perceive pain.

> A child's perception of pain appears to progress through the cognitive levels described by Piaget.[12]

Box 2.2 summarizes how children perceive pain at each of Piaget's stages of cognitive development.

Other studies have found that:

- younger children (four to six years) are more likely to attribute physical characteristics to their pain than older children (seven to 10 years)[17]

- the drawings (of pain) and coping strategies cited by children aged five to nine years focused on the physical aspects of pain; by the age of 11 years psychological coping strategies and depictions of pain of psychological origin appeared. At 13 years, 35% of coping strategies were psychological[18]

- a developmental trend was noted in the words used to describe pain; five year-olds used a total of five words to describe pain while 13 year-olds used 26 words[18]

- during the pre-operational stage (four to seven years) the child begins to use language to express pain. Although vocabulary may be limited and verbal reports of pain encounter validity and reliability problems, the child can now understand simple instructions. The changes are comparable with Piaget's stages of development[19]

- Gaffney and Dunne found an increasing use of semi-abstract ideas in children's definitions of pain, with a lessening of concrete definitions in a relationship with increasing age. They concluded that the changes corresponded to Piaget's stages of cognitive development.[20]

Children's perceptions of the cause and effect of pain develop as they mature. This maturation appears to parallel Piaget's stages of cognitive development.

Box 2.2 How children perceive the cause and effect of pain[12]

Piaget's stage of development	Perception of pain
Pre-operational (2–7 years)	Pain is primarily a physical experience
	Think about the magical disappearance of pain
	Not able to distinguish between cause and effect of pain
	Pain is often perceived as punishment for a wrong doing or bad thought[13] particularly if the child did something he or she was told not to do immediately before he or she started experiencing pain
	Children's egocentricity means that they hold someone else responsible for their pain and, therefore, are likely to strike out verbally or physically when they have pain
	Child is apt to tell a nurse who gave them an injection, 'You are mean'[14]
Concrete operational (7–11 years)	Relate to pain physically
	Able to specify location in terms of body parts
	Increased awareness of the body and internal organs means that fear of bodily harm is a strong influence in their perception of painful events
	Fear of total annihilation (body destruction and death) enters their thinking[15,16]
Transitional formal (10–12 years)	Have a perception of pain that is not quite as sophisticated as formal operational children
	Their perception of pain is not as literal as would be expected in children who are in the concrete operational stage of development

Box 2.2   Continued

Piaget's stage of development	Perception of pain
	Children in the transitional-formal stage were beginning to understand the concept of IF ... THEN propositions
Formal operational (12 years and above)	Begin to solve problems
	Do not always have required coping mechanisms to facilitate consistent mature responses
	Imagine the sinister implications of pain[3]

Reissland also found significant differences between the ability of younger children (four to seven years) and older children (seven to 13 years) to describe physical and cognitive coping strategies for pain. Younger children were also found to have fewer coping mechanisms and depended on their parents to cope for them.[21]

Nurses, therefore, need to encourage parents, particularly of younger children, to help their children cope with the pain they are experiencing. Many parents may never have seen their child in severe pain before so the nurse needs to help the parent identify ways in which they can help their children cope with the pain.[22] Parents can help their child in a number of ways which include:

- giving them a 'cuddle'
- using distraction methods such as reading a story.

'The fact that hospitalized children demonstrate less advanced notions of illness causality than healthy children is not fully understood but may be due to cognitive regression due to the stress and anxiety associated with acute illness or hospitalization.'[7]

'Cognitive regression may occur under distress, and children who are usually capable of logical thought may regress to using less mature thought processes and more fantasy.'[23]

Children's experiences of illness and hospitalization may affect their perception of, and their ability to cope with, pain. So in considering how children's understanding of the cause and effect of pain develops it is important to consider whether sick and/or hospitalized children experience any alteration in their perception of pain. Several studies have examined this area:

- Unrah et al. found that suffering from chronic pain may result in a child having a maturer perception of the cause and effect of pain than would normally be expected[24]

- Eiser states that although Piaget thought that sick children, because of their experiences, would have a more mature concept of illness, in fact the opposite appears to be true[25]

- McCaffery stated that studies have shown that frequent exposure to painful stimuli does not desensitize subjects but, instead, increases their sensitivity to the pain[14]

- contrary to common belief, children do not become accustomed to pain[26]

- under the stress of illness, regression to earlier modes of thinking may occur, with an associated decrease in a child's ability to verbalize about pain[20]

- children (aged nine to 12 years) who had been hospitalized described pain in a different way from children who had not been in hospital. Children who had been in hospital listed causes of pain that were related to illness and medical procedures more often than did non-hospitalized children.[27]

Health care professionals need to remember that children who have had repeated painful procedures may be more sensitive to pain than other children, and that their perception of pain may differ from the expected norm.

Pain differs from person to person, and culture to culture; individuals have their own unique pain threshold.[28,29]

Individuals differ in their responses to pain; as well as taking a child's level of cognitive development into account each child must have his or her perception of pain individually assessed.

Children's pain vocabulary

'Contrary to the widespread belief that children's pain descriptors are inadequate, almost 70% of the sample (n = 994) provided excellent single pain descriptors such as stabbing, burning, squeezing, jabbing, pressing, dull and agonizing. Furthermore a number of children (n = 286) were able to generate excellent descriptive sentences.'[30]

'Our data shows unequivocally that young children can provide a wealth of information about their pain experiences. Three procedural components are of crucial importance to obtaining such information. These are the type of question used, the child's perception of his role and capabilities, and the psychological climate of the interview setting.'[31]

A number of studies have demonstrated that children are able to describe their pain:

* children do spontaneously use descriptive words to describe the quality of their pain[32]

* Jerrett and Evans found that the majority of children responded spontaneously with a variety of adjectives, pain descriptors and phrases[33]

* Abu-Saad asked children aged nine to 15 years (n = 10) to describe their pain; the children used a total of 18 words to describe how their pain felt[34]

* it is possible to elicit the words used to describe pain from children using an appropriate interviewing technique[31]

* Gaffney states that all the studies carried out attest to children's familiarity with, and ability to talk about, pain, even as young as five years of age[35]

* Wilkie et al. developed a list of words known and used to describe pain by children, aged eight to 17 years, from a variety of ethnic backgrounds.[36]

A number of implications for nursing practice can be identified from the information presented in this chapter. They are summarized in Box 2.3.

Summary

* Children develop an understanding of illness and of the cause and effect of pain that reflects Piaget's stages of cognitive development.

Box 2.3 Implications for nursing practice

- Nurses need knowledge regarding children's level of development and their understanding of the cause and effect of pain

- Age-appropriate explanations about pain and treatment are required

- A *pre-operational child* needs reassurance that pain is not a punishment

- A *pre-operational child* may 'hate' the nurse who appears to be inflicting pain

- A *pre-operational child* cannot see the connection between treatment and relief of pain

- A *concrete operational* child needs reassurance about his/her fears regarding bodily annihilation

- A *concrete operational* child needs appropriate explanations about his/her pain and treatment

- A *formal operational* child needs opportunities to discuss his/her fears

- A *formal operational* child needs information about his/her condition and treatment

---

- Children as young as five years are able to talk about pain, although their vocabulary is different from that used by adults.[35]

- Perrin and Perrin found that physicians and nurses tend not to approach children according to their developmental level but instead address all children as if they are in the concrete operational stage. This can be seen to have implications for the quality of care provided.[2]

- Nurses, and other health care professionals, need to develop a knowledge base regarding children's level of understanding and incorporate this knowledge into their clinical practice.

- Nurses will then be in a position to provide the children they are caring for with a better quality of care; management and control of pain should also be improved.

- Until nurses, and other health care professionals, begin to consider routinely a child's developmental level when assessing pain, children will continue to suffer unnecessary pain.

References

1   Thompson KL and Varni JW (1986) A developmental cognitive-biobehavioral approach to pediatric pain assessment. *Pain.* **25**: 283–96.

2   Perrin EC and Perrin JM (1983) Clinicians' assessments of children's understanding of illness. *Am J Dis Child.* **137**: 874–8.

3   Muller DJ, Harris PJ and Wattley L (1986) *Nursing Children: Psychology, Research and Practice.* Harper & Rowe, London.

4   Bibace R and Walsh ME (1980) Development of children's concepts of illness. *Pediatrics.* **66** (6): 912–17.

5   Brewster AB (1982) Chronically ill hospitalised children's concepts of their illness. *Pediatrics.* **69**: 355–62.

6   Fieldman WS and Varni JW (1985) Conceptualisation of health and illness by children with spina bifida. *Child Health Care.* **13**: 102–8.

7   Perrin EC and Gerrity PS (1981) There's a demon in your belly: children's understanding of illness. *Pediatrics.* **67** (6): 841–9.

8   McGrath PA (1990) *Pain in Children: Nature, Assessment and Treatment.* The Guildford Press, New York.

9   Beales JG, Lennox Holt PJ, Keen JH and Mellor VP (1983) Children with juvenile chronic arthritis: their beliefs about their illness and therapy. *Ann Rheum Dis.* **42**: 481–6.

10 Yoos HL (1994) Children's illness concepts: old and new paradigms. *Pediatr Nurs.* **20** (2): 134–40, 145.

11 Haslam D (1969) Age and perception of pain. *Psychon Sci.* **15**: 86–7.

12 Hurley A and Whelan EG (1988) Cognitive development and children's perception of pain. *Pediatr Nurs.* **14** (1): 21–4.

13 Gildea JH and Quirk TR (1977) Assessing the pain experience in children. *Nurs Clin North Am.* **1**: 631–7.

14 McCaffery M (1972) *Nursing Management of the Patient with Pain.* Lippincott, Philadelphia.

15 Schultz NV (1971) How children perceive pain. *Nurs Outlook.* **3** (6): 670–3.

16 Alex JA and Ritchie MR (1992) School-aged children's interpretation of their experience with acute surgical pain. *Pediatr Nurs.* **7** (3): 171–80.

17 Scott R (1978) 'It hurts red': a preliminary study of children's perceptions of pain. *Percept Motor Skills.* **47**: 787–91.

18 Jeans ME and Gordan D (1981) *Developmental characteristics of the concept of pain.* Paper presented at the third world congress on pain, Edinburgh, Scotland.

19 Jeans ME (1983) The measurement of pain in children. In: *Pain Measurement and Assessment* (ed. R Melzack). Raven Press, New York.

20 Gaffney A and Dunne EA (1986) Developmental aspects of children's definitions of pain. *Pain.* **26**: 105–17.

21 Reissland N (1983) Cognitive maturity and the experience of fear and pain in hospital. *Soc Sci Med.* **17**: 1389–95.

22 Eland J (1985) The child who is hurting. *Semin Oncol Nurs.* **1** (2): 116–22.

23 Blos P (1978) Children think about illness: their concepts and beliefs. In: *Psychosocial Aspects of Pediatric Care* (ed. E Gellert). Grune & Stratton, New York.

24 Unrah A, McGrath P, Cunningham SJ *et al.* (1983) Children's drawings of their pain. *Pain.* **17**: 385–92.

25   Eiser C (1985) *The Psychology of Childhood Illness.* Springer-Verlag, New York.
26   Wong DL and Baker CM (1988) Pain in children: comparison of assessment scales. *Pediatr Nurs.* **14** (1): 9–17.
27   Savedra M, Gibbons P, Tesler M. Ward J and Wegner C (1982) How do children describe pain? A tentative assessment. *Pain.* **14**: 95–104.
28   Melzack R and Wall PD (1982) *The Challenge of Pain.* Penguin Books, Middlesex.
29   Sofaer B (1992) *Pain: A Handbook for Nurses.* (2nd edn) Chapman & Hall, London.
30   Ross DM and Ross SA (1984) Childhood pain: the school-aged child's viewpoint. *Pain.* **20**: 179–91.
31   Ross DM and Ross SA (1984) The importance of type of question, psychological climate and subject set in interviewing children about pain. *Pain.* **19**: 71–9.
32   Tesler MD, Savedra MC, Ward JA *et al.* (1989) Children's words for pain. In: *Management of Pain, Fatigue and Nausea* (eds SG Funk *et al.*). Macmillan, London.
33   Jerrett M and Evans K (1986) Children's pain vocabulary. *J Adv Nurs.* **11**: 403–8.
34   Abu-Saad H (1984) Assessing children's response to pain. *Pain.* **19**: 163–71.
35   Gaffney A (1993) Cognitive development aspects of pain in school-age children. In: *Pain in Infants, Children and Adolescents* (eds NL Schechter, CB Berde and M Yaster). Williams & Wilkins, Baltimore.
36   Wilkie DJ, Holzemer WL, Tesler MD *et al.* (1990) Measuring pain quality: validity and reliability of children's and adolescents' pain language. *Pain.* **41**: 151–9.

Further reading

Kister MC and Patterson CJ (1980) Children's conceptions of the causes of illness: Understanding of contagion and use of immanent justice. *Child Dev.* **51**: 839–46.

McGrath PJ and Craig KD (1989) Developmental and psychological factors in children's pain. *Pediatr Clin North Am.* **36** (4): 823–35.

Pidgeon V (1985) Children's concepts of illness: implications for health teaching. *MCN.* **14**: 23–35.

Rushworth H (1996) Nurses' knowledge of how children view health and illness. *Paediatr Nurs.* **8** (9): 23–7.

Whitt JK, Dykstra W and Taylor CA (1979) Children's conceptions of illness and cognitive development: implications for pediatric practitioners. *Clin Pediatr.* **18**: 327–35.

3 Pain pathways

Introduction

Someone may step on a nail and feel pain; another person may step on hot coals and feel nothing. How is this? Pain pathways are essential for life and yet they are flexible and able to learn. It is important, when treating pain, to understand the pathways and activity of pain fibres in order to comprehend the sites of action and effects of analgesics.

For a normal individual to sense pain, a nerve impulse must be initiated in nerve endings and pass along specific nerve fibres to the spinal cord. This impulse then passes up the spinal cord to specific areas of the brain responsible for the sensation of pain. It is similar to a letter being delivered by the Post Office; there are a number of different steps that must be followed for final delivery to occur.

Peripheral pain receptors

It is possible to sense pain all over the body both in the skin and as part of all tissues.

- There are no definite structures in the body that may be described specifically as pain receptors.

- Instead there are numerous branched free nerve endings of myelinated and unmyelinated neurones.

- These free nerve endings permeate the skin throughout the dermis and epidermis.

- The spread and number of these nerve endings correspond to the sensitivity of each area of skin to pain.

- These free nerve endings are termed nociceptors.

- In deep structures, such as cornea, dentine and periosteum, they are unimodal receptors responding only to pain.

- In the skin they are polymodal and respond to a number of stimulations such as heat, light touch, chemicals and pain.[1]

- Normally if the stimulus of these polymodal receptors is light then the sensation is perceived as touch or temperature; if the stimulus reaches a certain level then the sensation is one of pain. In chronic inflammation or in some chronic pain syndromes these receptors perceive any stimulus as pain.

The substances released by tissues in response to pain are also those released in response to tissue damage or distortion. They are:

- ions such as potassium and hydrogen

- histamine

- serotonin (5-hydroxytryptamine 5HT)

- prostaglandins and leukotrienes from the damaged tissues

- bradykinin from the circulation

- substance P from the free nerve endings.

The effects of these substances are variable. Bradykinin is, for example, able to initiate the pain sequence on its own but in order to increase the sensitivity of local structures it requires the presence of prostaglandins and/or 5HT.[2]

The result of this release of substances is to generate nerve impulses, to decrease the threshold for other local nerves to fire and increase the background activity of primary nerve fibres (*secondary hyperalgesia*). This results in a state of higher awareness for local nerve fibres.[3]

Non-steroidal anti-inflammatory drugs (NSAIDs) are active at nerve endings, inhibiting the production of prostaglandins. NSAIDs also indirectly inhibit the secondary hyperalgesic action of bradykinin. Thus NSAIDs act to inhibit the initial nerve impulse.[4] As there are a number of substances that act to generate nerve impulses it can be seen that NSAIDs will not produce complete analgesia.

Peripheral sensory nerves

- Nerve fibres are divided into three main groups by differences in structure and speed of impulse transmission – type A, B and C.

- Group A nerves have been further subdivided in terms of transmission speeds into Aα, Aβ, Aγ and Aδ nerves.

- All nerves that are responsible for the transmission of sensory impulses will produce the sensation of pain if they are stimulated sufficiently.

- Aδ and C fibres are, however, the two groups of nerves specifically responsible for the transmission of pain as a sensation.

- It is the free nerve endings of these fibres that are the nociceptors.

- Eighty per cent of pain impulses are carried in C fibres.

- The C fibres are unmyelinated and therefore slow. They are responsible for producing a sensation of pain that is aching, diffuse and uncomfortable.

- The Aδ fibres are myelinated, and therefore faster, producing pain that is sharp, discrete and immediate. The pattern of transmission along Aδ fibres can code for the intensity and character of the pain impulse.

The peripheral nerve is made up of groups of nerve fibres (or axons). They are arranged together in bundles. These bundles of nerve axons are covered by the protective outer layers of the nerve. In a mixed peripheral nerve the motor fibres are usually found along the outside of the nerve with the sensory fibres situated in the centre. This explains the onset of motor block before sensory block when local anaesthetics are applied to the nerve.

In the neonate the peripheral nerves are unmyelinated. The peripheral nerves are not completely myelinated until the third year of life, unlike nerves in the spinal cord, which are myelinated at birth. This was used until recently as a rationale to suggest that neonates are able to feel less pain than older children or adults.[5] However, myelination is not necessary for nerve transmission only for speed of transmission. The distance of nerve transmission in an adult is nearly 2 m from toe to brain; in the neonate it is closer to 50 cm. The shorter distances that the nerve impulses need to travel compensate for the lack of myelination. It is only with growth and the increased distance of nerve transmission that myelination of the nerves becomes necessary.

Peripheral nociceptive transmission

Nerves are *excitable structures*. At rest they are poised for action all of the time. This readiness is produced in the following way:

- in a nerve axon, molecules of sodium are actively expelled to the outside which increases the concentration of positively charged ions on the exterior of the cell

- to balance this, negatively charged ions would also move with the sodium ions to restore electrical neutrality

- these negative ions are, however, too large to pass through the membrane of the nerve axon, and thus a *potential difference* exists. This is usually in the order of -70 to -90 mV

- if the potential difference decreases towards zero the ability of nerve axons to expel the sodium ions is decreased

- if this trend towards zero continues, either by one large initiating stimulus (strong pain), or by the summation of many smaller pain impulses, the ability to expel sodium ions disappears and they flood into the cell

- this changes the electrical potential of the cell and a nerve impulse (the *action potential*) is generated

- once a nerve impulse is started, the change in electrical potential is transmitted along the whole of the cell to the nerve synapse in the spinal cord

- this nerve impulse may then be transmitted along a second nerve pathway but only if it produces enough change in electrical potential in the second axon to produce another action potential

- there are a number of primary fibres at the origin of the second nerve, some of which will excite the nerve and some of which will inhibit the nerve, thus allowing modulation of the nerve impulse.

Local anaesthetic agents act by inhibiting the movement of sodium into cells thus preventing the generation of the nerve impulse. They can, therefore, produce complete inhibition of the nerve impulse and, thus, complete analgesia and motor block of the area served by the individual nerve. The larger the size of the nerve blocked, the greater the extent of analgesia. For example, if the sciatic nerve in the upper thigh is blocked by local anaesthetic, then the whole of the limb below the knee is anaesthetized and unable to move.

To pass through the nerve membranes the local anaesthetic agents have to be un-ionized (i.e., lipid-soluble). In solution they exist in equilibrium between ionized and un-ionized forms. The degree of ionization depends on the local pH of the tissues. The lower the pH of the environment the more ionized they are, which means that local anaesthetics are less able to pass through tissues. In areas of inflammation, such as abscesses, the pH is low; local anaesthetic drugs cannot pass through the nerve membranes and are ineffective.

The transmission of nerve impulses in the spinal cord

If the peripheral nerves may be seen as telephone lines then the spinal cord is the first relay station. It is also the first filter removing unnecessary messages but also amplifying important ones.

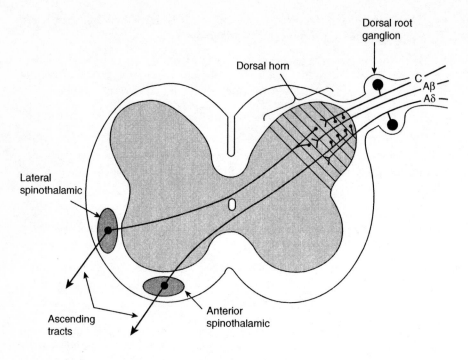

Figure 3.1: Pathways in the spinal cord.

- The afferent fibres arrive in the spinal cord via the dorsal horn, a collection of neurones and interneurones. They then divide into branches that go up or down the cord thus dissociating the nerve impulse (Figure 3.1).

- At each level of the cord there are discrete collections of neurones called laminae in the dorsal horn.

- Aδ fibres connect to laminae I, II and III and then cross the spinal cord to travel up the spinal cord in specific groups. These are called the spino-reticular and spinothalamic tracts (Figure 3.2). The transmission is thus retaining the fast speed of sensation from these nerves.

- The C fibres connect with the same laminae but also with a number of other neurones:
  - ascending tracts on the same side
  - interneurones to motor neurones and sympathetic neurones, resulting in spinal reflexes and sympathetic manifestations of acute and chronic pain
  - slow ascending tracts to various regions of the brain, resulting in a diffuse pain sensation.

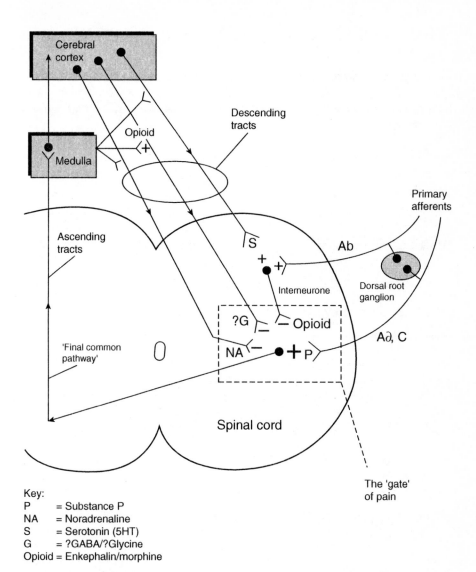

Figure 3.2: A schematic diagram of the central pain pathways.

- Aβ fibres terminate in the deeper laminae (IV–VII) and ascend in different tracts.

- There are interneurones between all laminae.

It can be seen, therefore, that there are two separate types of ascending pain transmission:

- sharp pain that travels via Aδ fibres, spinoreticular tracts, thalamus and sensory cortex

- diffuse pain, which travels via C fibres, spinoreticular tracts (among others), the reticular formation, the limbic system and the hypothalamus.

These pathways compete all the time to enable or prevent the pain stimulus.

Modulation of pain transmission in the spinal cord

As has been seen above, there are a large number of tracts that all pass through the spinal cord. For all of these tracts there are specific points in the spinal cord where the final decision is taken as to whether the stimulus passes to the brain or not. This forms the hypothesis of the *gate-control theory of pain* (Figure 3.2). This theory was first proposed by Melzack and Wall in 1965.[6]

- The gate-control theory is based on the fact that the pain sensation is transmitted by Aδ and C fibres to the spinal cord which synapse with ascending neurones for onward transmission to the brain. This is the normal state.

- However non-pain neurones (for example Aβ) can prevent the transmission of C fibre pain impulses by preventing synaptic transmission to ascending fibres (*closing the gate*), stopping pain sensation.

- Conversely, repeated stimulation by non-pain neurones of Aδ will amplify the pain impulse (*opening the gate*), increasing the intensity of pain sensation.

- The gate may also be closed by the descending pathways, decreasing the sensation of pain.

- This gate appears to be controlled by multisynaptic T (transmission) cells whose activity is dependent on the number of impulses it receives from inhibitory and excitatory fibres.

- A person's emotional or anxiety state can also close or open the gate.

It has recently been shown that the repetitive firing of C fibres will increase the excitability of neurones and interneurones in the spinal cord, thus reducing the threshold for transmission of pain and other sensations; this is described as *wind-up*.[7]

Neurotransmitters in the spinal cord

Substance P is the main neurotransmitter associated with diffuse pain, while glutamic acid is the transmitter for sharp pain. The phenomenon of wind-up is partly due to the interaction of two mediators: glutamic acid and N-methyl D-aspartate (NMDA), and substance P.[8]

- Opioids inhibit the release of substance P, by direct stimulation of opiate receptors (Figure 3.2), therefore, inhibiting neurotransmitters.

- Adrenaline inhibits the release of substance P.

- Ketamine is thought to act by both adrenaline-type receptors and also by preventing the amplification of pain that is present with inflammatory responses.[9]

- Transcutaneous electrical nerve stimulation (TENS), acupuncture and cold increase the frequency of transmission of Aβ fibres; the gate is closed and less pain is sensed in the brain.

Supraspinal pathways

There are four regions of the brain that act as second relay sites.

Reticular formation

Nerves from the spinoreticular tract synapse here, and tertiary nerves both ascend to the cortex and descend to the spinal cord (Figure 3.2). The reticular formation is important for other non-painful stimuli and is thought to be important in the sleep/awake state. It may be that this region produces a higher awareness when painful stimuli are present.

Limbic system

Another system for nerve modulation. This region is also important for benzodiazepine receptors and is probably associated with the feelings of anxiety associated with pain.

Thalamus

The final relay before the cerebral cortex. It is capable of the crude interpretation of pain and is the final site of pain modulation.

Cerebral cortex

Pain is sensed in this region at the site of the post-central gyrus.

Modulation of nerve transmission above the spinal cord

Electrical stimulation of the periaqueductal grey matter (in the midbrain) produces a descending inhibition of pain transmission identical to the effect of introducing morphine to the spinal cord. The pathways are corticothalamic pathways, raphe nuclei and descending posterior trunks of the spinal cord. The transmitter in these pathways is thought to be 5HT although there are also opioid receptors involved. Opioid receptors are also important in the reticular formation and limbic system, resulting in sedation and decreased anxiety. Although the structures are supraspinal, the actual modulation occurs at the synapse of the descending pathways, that is the level of the spinal cord, opening or closing the gate.

Ways in which the transmission of pain stimuli can break down

It is important to remember that because the transmission of the nerve impulse is dependent on a number of nerves, varying in type, purpose and effects, the nervous system can be modified at a number of different sites. It is easy to imagine that the system could break down.

- The descending pathways could be damaged resulting in the continuing transmission of pain impulses to the brain, producing chronic pain. Using the analogy of the post office, everybody's mail is delivered to you.

- The connections between the spinal cord and the sympathetic nerves could be damaged, resulting in sympathetic dystrophies that accompany chronic pain. There are no recordings that the mail has been delivered.

- The loss of a limb does not change the descending pathways or spinal reflexes that would normally modulate nerve impulses from the limb. The brain thinks that the limb is still attached, resulting in 'phantom limb' pain. Receiving imaginary mail.

Developmental considerations

Neonates

The neonate does not have all of these pathways present at the same time. The first pathway to mature is the C fibre type 'slow' pain. The neonate will give a graded response, dependent on the intensity of the pain stimulus. There are no methods of modulation. After the age of 30 weeks there is some degree of learning in the pain system; the nerves are able to demonstrate decreased responsiveness after repeated stimulation.[10] The ability to discriminate the site of the nerve impulse only becomes available after myelination of the nerves; this is complete in the spinal cord after 30 weeks of gestation. The body is then able to learn and react to various stimuli, becoming a more dynamic system.

The slow maturation of the descending systems means that when neonates feel pain they are only able to react in a general, explosive manner with manifestations such as withdrawal, crying and grimacing.

Infants

In the first year of life, after about three months of age, the infant is able to localize pain and produce specific reactions of protection and withdrawal of the injured site.[11] The responses of crying and facial expression remain the commonest modalities for the expression of pain. There are also signs of social changes, with acute pain resulting in general withdrawal, sleep disorders and loss of appetite.

Older children

Pre-school children are characterized by their ability to talk and discuss their pain although their ability to communicate is limited. Pain is described in terms of absolutes; it is either really intense or non-existent. The intensity of pain at this age depends more on environmental changes, with parental presence being of prime importance. From the age of about five to seven years, children become more adult in their expression of pain. They are able to describe pain in terms of previous pain experience, severity and type of pain. Children's understanding of the cause of pain at this age, however, has not reached the level of adult understanding. (*See* Chapter 2 for further discussion of children's cognitive level and their perception of pain.)

Summary

- When treating pain it is important to understand the pathways and activity of pain fibres in order to comprehend the sites of action and effects of analgesic drugs.
- Pain 'receptors' are present all over the body.
- Chemicals are released by tissues in response to pain.
- The release of these chemicals generates the nerve impulse.
- Two groups of nerve fibres are specifically responsible for pain transmission: Aδ and C fibres.
- The spinal cord acts as the first relay for transmission of pain stimuli.
- A large number of tracts pass through the spinal cord; for all of these there are specific points in the spinal cord where the final decision is taken as to whether the stimulus passes to the brain or not.
- This forms the basis of the gate-control theory of pain.
- Analgesics act at specific receptors, but at different sites, resulting in synergistic activity. The use of a combination of analgesics is thus advocated.

References

1   Burgess PR and Perl ER (1967) Myelinated afferent fibres responding specifically to noxious stimulation of the skin. *J Physiol London*. **190**: 541–62.
2   Dray A (1995) Inflammatory mediators in pain. *Br J Anaesth*. **75** (2): 125–31.
3   Raja S, Meyer JN and Meyer RA (1988) Peripheral mechanisms of somatic pain. *Anesthesiology*. **68**: 571–90.
4   Moncada S and Vane JR (1979) Mode of action of aspirin drugs. *Adv Intern Med*. **24**: 1–22.
5   Shearer MH (1986) Surgery of the paralysed, unanaesthetized newborn. *Birth*. **13**: 79–81.
6   Melzack R and Wall PD (1965) Pain mechanism – a new theory. *Science*. **150**: 971–9.

7   Urban L, Thompson SW, Nag I et al. (1994) Hyperexcitability in the spinal dorsal horn: co-operation of neuropeptides and excitation amino acids. In: *Cellular Mechanisms of Sensory Processing* (ed. L Urban). Springer-Verlag, Berlin, pp. 379–99.
8   Woolf CJ (1989) Recent advance in the pathophysiology of acute pain. *Br J Anaesth.* **63**: 139–46.
9   Edwards ND, Fletcher A, Cole JR et al. (1993) Combined infusions of morphine and ketamine for postoperative pain in elderly patients. *Anaesth.* **48**: 124–7.
10 Anand KJS and Hickey PR (1987) Pain and its effects in the human neonate and fetus. *N Engl J Med.* **317**: 1321–9.
11 Barr RG (1982) Pain tolerance and developmental changes in pain perception. In: *Developmental-Behavioral Pediatrics* (eds MD Levine, WB Carey, AC Crocker and RT Gross). Saunders, Philadelphia, pp. 505–12.

Further reading

Clancy J and McVicar A (1992) Subjectivity of pain. *Br J Nurs.* **1** (1): 8–12.

Davis P (1993) Opening up the gate control theory. *Nurs Standard.* **7** (45): 25–7.

Jacques A (1994) Physiology of pain. *Br J Nurs.* **3** (12): 607–10.

Jessop J (1993) Basic neurophysiology of pain. *Curr Anaesth Crit Care.* **4**: 64–9.

Wall PD and Melzack R (1989) *Textbook of Pain.* Churchill Livingstone, London.

4 Quality and pain management

Introduction

Health care professionals need to examine the role quality can play in achieving effective pain management.

Quality is a central issue in nearly every professional organization.[1]

Over recent years there has been an increasing interest in quality in public services with an emphasis on addressing the wishes of the users.[2]

This chapter will examine how quality can be incorporated into the management of pain in children, and the benefits this brings to the child and family. It will give a definition of quality and will discuss how a quality system for pain can be implemented. Finally ways of organizing a pain management audit will be identified.

What is quality?

No single definition of quality encompasses all that the word implies, but quality clearly has some attributes of excellence, involving the right things for the job and is to do with getting things right first time.[3]

- Quality is a difficult concept to define and encompasses a variety of different aspects.

- Quality is accompanied by concepts such as service, customer orientation and effectiveness.[1]

- Quality is the extent to which services meet the customer's needs.[4]

- Quality, to the customer, is determined by the degree to which the product satisfies the need for which it was acquired.[5]

> Whatever definition or concept of quality is used, the vital factor is how to put it into practice.[2]

- As we approach the 21st century, quality within the health care system in the UK is becoming increasingly important.
- Health care professionals need to ensure that improvements become reality.
- Quality needs to focus on all aspects of service delivery, and pain management must be included within this framework.

The effective management of pain is a challenge facing all health care professionals. The implementation of a quality strategy can help establish the systems needed to manage children's pain.

Implementing a quality system for pain management

> Many hospitals have written measurable standards of care and service.[6]
>
> This is an essential component if success is to be achieved in implementing a quality-driven pain service.

To make any real impact on service delivery, standards must be easily transferable into the care setting and have meaning and ownership by staff. Koch describes several key characteristics that are essential to facilitate real service development:[6]

- all groups of staff must have standards
- the standards need to be understood by all staff
- the standards need to be monitored at either local level or management level
- the standard setting and monitoring process needs to benefit the patient.

To achieve a quality-driven service in pain management, it is essential for the organization to be fully committed to these key characteristics and for individuals within the workplace to be actively involved in the setting of standards.

The first step in establishing a quality system for pain management is to establish a working party comprising staff who have an interest in pain management from across the multi-disciplinary team. This group should:

- set out clear terms of reference with identified goals and time scales

- set up a formal communication channel within the organization and throughout management

- write a standard of care for pain management

- this standard should be measurable

- an audit criteria should be written so that it is possible to establish whether the standard of care is being achieved.

> Once formal standards are set, quality auditing and monitoring is an essential component of a quality management system.

Once the standard has been written, an initial audit should be carried out. Areas where improvements in care are needed can then be identified. The pain working party can then prioritize these areas and write an action plan. The action plan should set out the steps needed to establish a quality pain management service and should be made up of achievable steps. Areas where improvements may be needed can be seen in Box 4.1.

Box 4.1   Steps that can be taken to improve the quality of pain management

- The use of a pain assessment tool

- Standardization of analgesic drugs

- Increasing the use of psychological/non-drug methods

- Education about pain management

- Writing a clinical protocol for pain management (see Chapter 8)

- Minimizing the use of intra-muscular injections

- Establishing a network of link nurses

- Writing information leaflets for the child and parents

- Identifying the need for a clinical nurse specialist

It is necessary to prioritize the steps which need to be taken and to be realistic about the length of time needed to implement change. Time needs to be allowed for staff training prior to implementing change.

The standard should be audited at three-monthly intervals providing an indication of the level of improvement. It is important for the pain working party to re-evaluate its action plan each time the standard is audited and re-prioritize the steps to be taken. To ensure that the care provided to the child and family is of the highest level, the action plan should be reviewed in the light of research in order to provide care which is evidence-based.

The establishment of communication channels throughout the organization is essential in managing change.[7] Quality is everyone's responsibility and there-fore it is important to gain commitment and motivation from others working within the organization.[2] McCarthy and Hicks discuss how essential it is to reassure staff that the system will:[3]

- be practical and workable

- allow for change, adaptation and development

- cope with unexpected circumstances

- belong to staff.

Pain relief is still not a priority among many health care professionals, result-ing in children suffering unnecessary pain (*see* Chapter 1). For parents and children pain is a priority; pain is often what causes them to seek medical advice. It is necessary, when striving to provide a quality service, to seek the views of the children and their parents with regard to the management of pain. When doing this:

- the information gathered must be accurate and reliable and acted upon

- the information must be a true representation of practice.

Quality management is about removing the reasons for problems, and not about solving or accommodating the same problems over and over again.[3]

- As health care professionals we have to provide the children in our care and their families with a communication channel to inform us of their perceptions of the service offered.

- This allows us to reflect on future developments within the service.

- Ways need to be established to find out the views of parents and children.

Brown outlines a variety of communication channels that can be used for the customer (parents and children) to talk to an organization:[8]

- feedback systems
- questionnaires
- customer clinics
- suggestion forms.

It would be possible, for example, to attach a short questionnaire to an information leaflet for parents or to have suggestion forms available for parents and children to complete.

To gain an accurate audit of quality it is essential that health care professionals use some of these methods to gain the child's and family's views about the service we offer and deliver. The method must be user friendly.

There are many innovative approaches to analysing the information gathered when the views of customers (parents and children) are sought. One method is the use of *quality circles* where a small group meets regularly and identifies, analyses and seeks solutions to work-related problems. A wide selection of pain issues could be discussed and solutions identified, in order to ensure a quality-driven service. This could be seen as part of the remit of the pain working party.

Children continue to suffer unnecessary pain.[9] Ensuring that this no longer happens requires a multi-dimensional approach; implementing a quality strategy is an essential part of this.

Summary

- Quality is about meeting the customer's needs.
- Implementation of a quality strategy can help establish the systems needed to manage children's pain effectively.
- Standards of care are an essential component of a quality strategy.
- A multi-disciplinary team needs to be established.
- After an initial audit of the standard of care, an action plan should be drawn up.
- The management of change needs to be considered.
- Communication channels need to be established.
- The views of children and parents should be considered.

References

1   Mastenbroek W (1991) *Managing for Quality in the Service Sector*. Blackwell, Oxford.
2   Audit Commission (1993) *Putting Quality on the Map. Measuring and Appraising Quality in the Public Service*. Occasional Paper No. 18, March. HMSO, London.
3   McCarthy J and Hicks B (1991) Quality in health care: application of the ISO 9000 standard. *Int J Health Care Quality Assurance*. **4** (4): 21–6.
4   Brant S (1991) Hearing the patient's story. *Int J Health Care Quality Assurance*. **5** (6): 5–7.
5   Webb I (1991) *Quest for Quality*. Industrial Society Press, London.
6   Koch H (1991) Quality of care and service. *Managing Service Quality*. **July**: 263–7.
7   Lancaster J and Lancaster W (eds) (1982) *The Nurse as a Change Agent*. CV Mosby, St Louis.
8   Brown A (1991) *Customer Care Management*. Butterworth-Heinemann, Oxford.
9   Cummings EA, Reid GJ, Finley A *et al.* (1996) Prevalence and source of pain in pediatric inpatients. *Pain*. **68**: 25–31.

5   Pain assessment in children

Introduction

Determining the level of pain a person may be experiencing is one of the most common and most difficult tasks for nurses to accomplish.[1]

The measurement of pain in children is a major challenge to health care professionals.[2]

Knowing how much pain a child is experiencing is the first step towards offering appropriate treatment for his or her pain.[3]

In order to manage pain in children, it is essential that a reliable, valid and measurable assessment is performed on a regular basis. This assessment should, ideally, take place before the child is in pain as well as during painful episodes, although this may be difficult for children admitted as emergencies, and should monitor the effect of any pharmacological and non-drug methods of treating pain. The assessment of pain also needs to be appropriate for the individual child and his or her family. This chapter will, therefore, start by examining how perceptions, beliefs and tolerance to pain differ between individual children. A number of pain assessment tools will also be reviewed, non-verbal behavioural clues will be identified, physiological indications of pain will be discussed, and guidelines for the effective management of pain provided. The problems of assessing pain in pre-verbal children and the pain assessment tools available for use in this group of children are discussed in Chapter 6.

Influences on children's pain

Each child will feel pain of differing levels and degrees and react to and cope with this in his or her own way.[4]

Individuals have their own unique pain threshold.[5]

There are many different influences on children's pain which are listed in Box 5.1. (How cognitive development affects a child's perception of pain was discussed in Chapter 2.)

Box 5.1   Influences on children's pain

- Developmental stage
- Culture
- Gender
- Personality
- Family
- Society
- Religion
- Previous experiences of pain

Culture

- British children tend to be stoical about their pain.
- Italian children tend to be more depressed and honest about their pain and concerned that they should be given immediate relief from their pain.[6] However, they forget their suffering once the pain has been removed.[7]
- Irish people are stoical about their pain but may be more concerned about the future consequences of their pain.[7]
- Kikuyu and Masai men are expected to be quiet and dignified about their pain but women are permitted to cry out or act in any way they please.[8]
- In the African Luo tribe, men are allowed to wail when in pain.[8]
- Most British children prefer to have company when they are in pain.[7]
- Australian children prefer to be on their own.[7]

These are just a few examples of cultural differences that exist in relation to pain; it must be remembered that children from the same culture will have their own differences. Cultural differences are evident in the way that children tolerate pain. The nurse's own culture will also affect his or her perception of a child's pain.[9]

Gender

It has been suggested that boys should be able to tolerate pain better than girls. However, in the author's experience on a children's orthopaedic ward there seems to be very little difference in the way that girls and boys tolerate their pain, although they may express it differently, for example, older girls cry more than older boys.[10] This is probably because there is a cultural expectation that 'big boys don't cry.'[10] Boys in a Western culture are expected to be strong and brave; girls are expected to be weaker and are allowed to express themselves.[7]

Personality

In laboratory tests extroversion has been associated with higher pain tolerance and introversion with a greater sensitivity to pain. Introverts, however, may complain less.[6]

Family and society influences

- Families pass on beliefs, traditions and customs.[7]

- If a member of a family has had a similar experience to his or her child, that individual might influence how well the child copes.

- This could become a vicious circle of anxiety and pain; 'pain increases anxiety and anxiety increases pain perception'.[12]

- As children mature they take on values from peers and teachers which may cause conflict with family values.[7]

- Society has clear expectations about 'appropriate' pain behaviour.[13]

Religion

- Children's religious beliefs will have an impact on their perception or tolerance of pain. For example, Jews seek help, sympathy and second opinions.[6,14]

- Hindus associate pain with karma (a burden from a previous pain incarnation).[7]

- Some Christians may see pain as a punishment for sin.[12]
- Other Christians believe that God allows pain but will enable them to cope with it.[12]

Previous experiences of pain

- Nurses feel that they can empathize with people in pain if they have suffered pain themselves, but they tend to judge someone's pain according to their own beliefs and values.[7]
- Nurses who have experienced considerable pain may overemphasize another's pain; the reverse may also be true.
- A child's previous experiences of pain alters his or her perception of pain.[15]
- Infants cry in anticipation during subsequent visits to immunization clinics.[16]

Children's previous experiences with pain will affect how they react to subsequent painful events.

> Children cope differently with pain; sound nursing judgement is needed to ensure accurate interpretation of their pain experience.[17]

Why assess pain?

- Unrelieved pain has a number of undesirable consequences (see Chapter 1).[18]
- Knowing how much pain children are experiencing is the first step towards offering appropriate treatment for their pain.[3]
- Accurate pain assessment provides an information base on which to provide effective pain management.[9]
- Without methods to assess pain quantitatively in children, it is impossible to plan appropriate interventions and their effectiveness.[19]

Pain should be assessed in order to intervene appropriately to control and manage the pain. Pain assessment should also be used to evaluate the effectiveness of pharmacological and non-drug interventions.

How to assess pain

The QUESTT tool encompasses many of the important features of pain assessment.[20]

Question the child

Use pain rating scales

Evaluate behaviour and physiological changes

Secure parents' involvement

Take the cause of pain into account

Take action and evaluate results

Question the child

- Ideally this should happen before any painful episodes occur.
- Discover any past experiences of pain.
- Are there any specific words used for pain?
- What is the child's perception of pain?
- What are the family's beliefs about pain?
- Involving the child in his or her pain management increases self-esteem which indirectly decreases their perception of pain.[21]

Use pain rating scales

- Each clinical area should have two or three pain assessment tools.
- Allow the child to choose an appropriate scale.
- Explain the use of the tool to the child.
- Pain assessment tools enable the nurse to acquire rapidly a clear perspective on a child's pain.[22]

Evaluate behaviour and physiological changes

- Observing the child's non-verbal clues is an important part of pain assessment; children do not always tell the truth about their pain.[23]

- Physiological changes in pulse and blood pressure can, in acute pain, be useful indicators that a child is in pain.[24]

- Physiological indicators should be used in conjunction with other methods of assessing pain.

Secure parents' involvement

- Discover how much or how little the parents would like to be involved in their child's pain assessment.

- Parents' involvement should not be taken for granted.

- Nurses often think that parents are the best people to assess their child's pain but parents may be stressed and may have little experience of seeing their child in pain.[23]

- Parents expect the nurse to know when their child is in pain.[23]

Take the cause of pain into account

- Health care professionals should have some knowledge of different conditions and the type and amount of pain that results.

- Acute pain should be assessed quickly and effectively.[25]

- Chronic pain assessment should be more relaxed with more time allowed for communication.[25]

Take action and evaluate results

- Give analgesics.

- Evaluate the effect of analgesics using a pain assessment tool.

For a child in chronic pain a different approach to assessing pain may be needed. Box 5.2 suggests some useful questions that can be used when assessing chronic pain in older children.

> **Box 5.2**   Questions that can be used when assessing chronic pain in older children (adapted from Schofield)[25]
>
> • Identify the exact location(s) of the pain
>
> • Establish the cause of the pain
>
> • Identify any aggravating or alleviating factors
>
> • What does the pain mean to the child?
>
> • Do they understand the cause or reason for the pain?
>
> • What coping strategies do they use?
>
> • What effect does the pain have on their life?

General principles of pain assessment

Assessment should be a continuous process and the methods that are used should enable the accurate evaluation of nursing interventions as well as suggesting changes in these interventions.[3]

• When assessing pain, record its frequency, duration and intensity on a flow chart.[26]

• Children may be unwilling to discuss their pain, for fear of the consequences, so assume the pain is present unless there is evidence that it is absent.[9]

• Using a pain rating scale ask the child how much pain he or she has.

• Involve the parents in the pain assessment.

• Evaluate physiological and behavioural clues.

• Reassess the child's pain rating having given time for pain-relieving interventions to take effect.

Ways of measuring children's pain

Pain can be measured by:

- behaviour (what children do)
- biological markers (how their bodies react)
- self-report (what children say).[27]

Non-verbal pain behaviours (what children do)

Children do not always tell the truth about their pain.[23,28] When assessing pain it is, therefore, important to observe their non-verbal clues. Non-verbal pain behaviours in children are identified in Box 5.3.

Box 5.3   Non-verbal assessment of pain in children

General behaviours	Specific behaviours
Changed behaviour	Banging head
Irritability	Pulling ear
Flat effect	Curling up on side
Unusual posture	Refusal to move limbs
Screaming	Constantly rubbing specific region
Reluctance to move	
Aggressiveness	
Increased clinging	
Unusual quietness	
Loss of appetite	
Restlessness	
Whimpering	
Sobbing	
Lying 'scared stiff'	
Lethargy	
Disturbed sleep pattern	

Physiological signs (how their bodies react)

- Most useful when combined with other data about pain-involving behaviours and pain-producing pathology.[18]

- If pain persists over a period of time there is less increase in the sympathetic responses. This phenomenon is known as adaptation.[29]

- These signs are used inappropriately by nurses at times when adaptation (to pain) could have been expected to have occurred.[30,31]

Physiological signs should not be used as the sole mechanism for assessing pain.

Assessment tools (what children say)

> The introduction of appropriate tools of measurement into clinical practice creates a vision of a systematic approach to the measurement of pain – a system in which personal beliefs, attitudes and subjectivity are reduced to a minimum.[32]

There are a number of pain assessment tools available for use in clinical practice that enable a systematic approach to be taken to pain assessment and measurement. The use of a pain assessment tool improves pain control and aids nursing care.[33] A list of some of the tools available can be seen in Box 5.4.

Using pain assessment tools

The selection of a pain assessment tool should be based on the child's age and cognitive ability, the time available to educate the child about the scale, and the knowledge nurses have about the scale.[34]

Visual analogue scale (Figure 5.1)

- Usually a 10 cm horizontal or vertical line with a mark at either end with 'no pain' on the left and 'worst pain imaginable' on the right.[25]

- The child marks the position along the line which may be measured with a ruler so that the measurement can be recorded on a chart.

- The child's own words could be substituted at either end.[9]

> **Box 5.4**   Examples of pain assessment tools available for use in clinical practice
>
> - Visual analogue scale
> - Verbal graphic rating scale
> - Numerical rating scale
> - Pain thermometer
> - Poker chip tool
> - Eland Color Scale
> - PATCh
> - Diaries
> - McGill Pain Questionnaire
> - Varni–Thompson Questionnaire
> - Faces scales

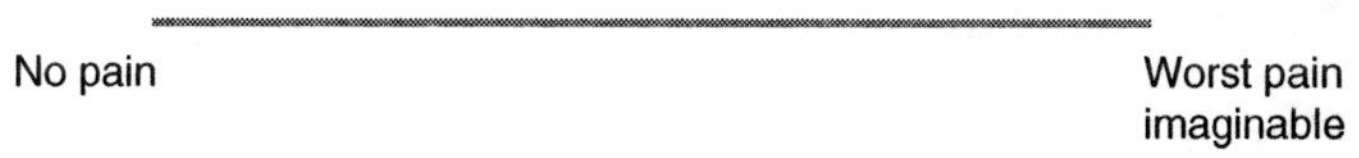

No pain   Worst pain
                                                                       imaginable

Figure 5.1:   Visual analogue scale.

- Useful for children with limited language skills but the child needs the cognitive ability to translate experience into analogue format and to be able to understand proportionality.[35]

Verbal graphic rating scale

A horizontal or vertical 10 cm line with descriptors written along the line starting at the left with 'no pain' to 'worst possible pain' on the right.[25]

Numerical rating scale

- A 10 cm line with 'no pain' on the far left and 'worst possible pain' on the far right line and numbered 0–10 or 0–5.

- Useful for assessing pain relief but children need to be numerate, which excludes most children under five years.[11]

Pain thermometer

Described as a vertical form of the numerical rating scale numbered 0–10 or 0–100.[36]

Poker chip tool[9]

- Four poker chips are placed in front of the child and described as *pieces of hurt*:

   - first chip – 'just a little hurt'

   - second chip – 'a little more hurt'

   - third chip – 'more hurt'

   - fourth chip – 'the most hurt you can have'.

Eland Color Scale (Figure 5.2)

- Provides information on the child's level of pain and the location of the pain.[9]

- Consists of two body outlines – the back and front of a child.

- There are four boxes titled 'no pain/hurt' to 'severe pain/worst hurt'.

- The child is given eight coloured pens and asked to choose four colours with which to colour on the boxes.

- Eland suggests providing yellow, orange, red, green, blue, purple, brown and black.[23]

- Each time children are assessed they colour the area on the body outline in the appropriate colours.

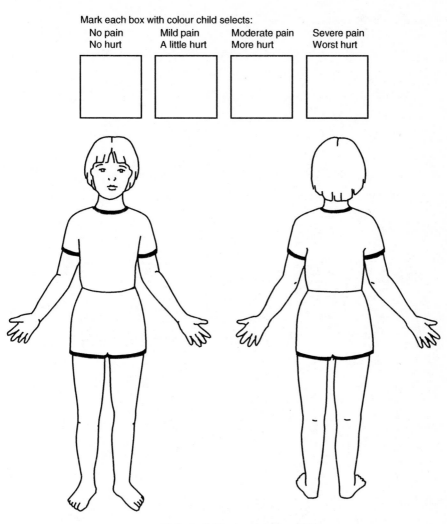

Mark each box with colour child selects:

| No pain | Mild pain | Moderate pain | Severe pain |
| No hurt | A little hurt | More hurt | Worst hurt |

(Indicate child's use of right and left)

Figure 5.2: Eland Color Scale

• Young children are able to locate their pain but it is useful to go through body parts with them to discover their knowledge of the body parts and left and right.[11]

• Studies have shown that young children are able to point on a body outline; the location of the pain was consistent with the child's diagnosis.[11]

• Children's choice of colour is not always consistent.[19]

Pain Assessment Tool for Children (PATCh) (Figure 5.3)

- Uses elements from five existing pain scales:[37]
  - faces
  - body outline
  - numerical visual analogue scale
  - descriptive words
  - behavioural scale

- Can be used at any age

- PATCh has been found to be reliable for children and nurses by the authors.

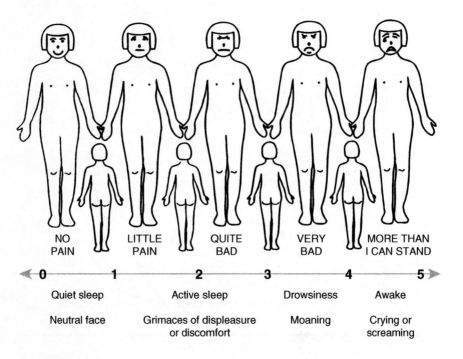

Figure 5.3: Pain Assessment Tool for Children (PATCh).

Diaries

- Particularly useful in the assessment of chronic pain.

- Can include a numerical rating scale and verbal descriptors.[35]

- Useful for children to explore their experience of pain and enable them to document any episodes of pain.[9]
- May result in children focusing on their pain more than they want.

McGill Pain Questionnaire[38]

- Aims to measure the qualities of pain.[25]
- Available in a shorter form and in many different languages.[38]
- Some of the questionnaires have a body outline so pain can be indicated.
- It is more appropriate for adolescents suffering chronic pain.[39]
- Takes a long time to complete and its usefulness is debatable.[40]

Varni–Thompson Questionnaire[41]

- Uses a body outline and visual analogue scale.[9]
- Has three components: child, adolescent and parent.
- Originally developed for chronic pain.
- Includes information on sensory, affective and evaluative components of the pain experience, location and intensity.

Faces scales

There are several faces scales. The following are the most commonly used:

Wong and Baker Faces Rating Scale[19] (Figure 5.4)

- For use with children aged three to 18 years.
- There are six faces numbered 0–5 depicting smiling to neutral to total misery.

Figure 5.4: Wong and Baker Faces Rating Scale.

- Explain to the child that the smiling face is smiling because it has no pain at all and that the crying face is crying because it has as much pain as it could possibly have.

- It is important to emphasize to children that they do not have to be crying for their pain to be represented by the crying face; it is how they feel 'inside'.

Bieri et al.*'s faces pain scale*[2] (Figure 5.5)

- Has 'superior scaling properties'.

- Simple, quick and easy to learn; children as young as three years have understood it.

- Faces derived from children's drawings.

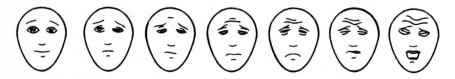

Figure 5.5:   The faces pain scale.

The Oucher[42] (Figure 5.6)

- Measures pain intensity in children aged three to 12 years.[9]
- Made up of two scales:
  - six photographs arranged vertically
  - a vertical numerical scale from 0–100.
- The scale of 0–100 means that a child needs to be able to count to 100 in order to use it.

Which scale should be used when?

None of the scales described is applicable for children of all ages. Box 5.5 suggests approximate ages for some of the more commonly used scales. (The assessment of pre-verbal children is discussed in Chapter 6.)

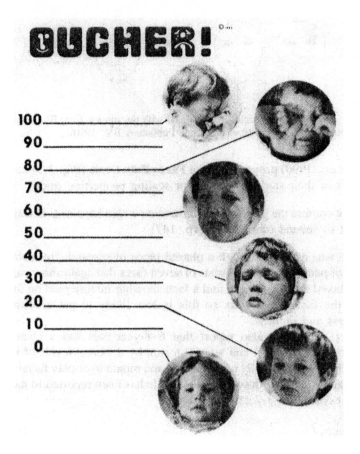

Figure 5.6:   The Oucher.

Validity and reliability of scales

> The wholesale adoption of such tools without careful analysis may not always lead to better practice.[3]
>
> For post-operative children many of the pain measurement systems are still being evaluated.[43]

For a pain assessment tool to measure a child's pain effectively it must be reliable and valid.

Box 5.5   Which tool should be used when?

Tool	Age group
Faces	From 3 years
Poker chips	4–8 years
Eland Color Scale	4–10 years
Numerical	From 9–10 years
Verbal Graphic Rating Scale	9–15 years
Oucher	3–12 years
	Useful with young children and those with language difficulties

Reliability

- Reliability refers to the consistency, stability and repeatability of measurements.[44]

- To ascertain that an instrument is capable of producing reliable data individuals in different groups, different settings and at different times must respond similarly.[45]

Validity

- Validity refers to the appropriateness, applicability and representativeness of using measurements as a 'true' finding.[46]

Oppenheim uses a clock to illustrate the difference between validity and reliability.[47] A clock is *valid* if it measures 'true' time and *reliable* if it does so consistently. A clock that is always 10 minutes slow is reliable but it would be invalid as it shows the wrong time. If it is sometimes slow and sometimes fast it is both unreliable and invalid.

Many of the pain assessment tools described require further studies to establish validity and reliability. A number of the studies that have been carried out have been conducted by the authors of the tools themselves and one wonders whether there was an element of bias in their findings. Meinhart and McCaffery, however, concluded that none of the tools were better than any other.[48]

> **Box 5.6** Guidelines for the management of pain in children (adapted from Gillies)[49]
>
> - Treat each child individually
> - Consider whether the pain has been effectively assessed
> - Observe non-verbal and physiological clues
> - Give prescribed analgesics
> - Use pharmacological and non-drug methods
> - If the child remains distressed consider whether the cause is still pain
> - If communication is unclear give the child the benefit of the doubt and treat distress as pain
> - If the child is still in pain, ask medical staff about using other drugs

Management of pain in children

Having assessed pain in children, it is important to intervene in order to control and manage the pain. Some guidelines for pain management in children are given in Box 5.6.

Summary

- Determining the level of pain a child may be experiencing is one of the most common and most difficult tasks for nurses to accomplish.[1]
- To manage pain in children a reliable, valid and measurable assessment should be performed on a regular basis.
- There are many different influences on children's pain including culture, gender, developmental stage and previous experiences of pain.
- Children cope with pain in different ways; pain is an individual phenomenon.
- Pain should be assessed in order to intervene to control and manage the pain.
- Pain assessment should evaluate the effectiveness of pharmacological and non-drug interventions.

- The QUESTT approach encompasses the important aspects of pain assessment.

- Assessment should be a continuous process and the methods that are used should enable the accurate evaluation of nursing interventions as well as suggesting changes in these interventions.[3]

- Pain can be measured by behaviour (what children do), biological markers (how their bodies react), and self-report (what children say).[27]

- Pain assessment tools need to be valid and reliable; further research is required in this area.

- Different tools need to be chosen for children of different ages.

- When assessing pain its frequency, duration and intensity should be recorded on a flow chart.

References

1   Bradshaw C and Zeanah PD (1986) Pediatric nurses' assessments of pain in children. *Pediatr Nurs.* **1** (5): 314–22.
2   Bieri D, Reeve RA, Champion GD *et al.* (1990) The Faces Pain Scale for the self-assessment of the severity of pain experienced by children: development, initial validation and preliminary investigation for ratio scale properties. *Pain.* **41**: 139–50.
3   Price S (1994) Assessing children's pain. *Br J Nurs.* **3** (20): 1046–8.
4   Adler S (1990) Taking children at their word: pain control in paediatrics. *Profession Nurse.* **May**: 398–401.
5   Sofaer B (1992) *Pain: a handbook for nurses.* (2nd edn) Chapman & Hall, London.
6   Zborowski M (1952) Cultural components in response to pain. *J Social Issues.* **8**: 16–30.
7   East E (1992) How much does it hurt? *Nurs Times.* **88** (40): 48–9.
8   Ngugi EN (1986) Pain: an African perspective. *Nurs Practice.* **1**: 169–76.
9   Carter B (1994) *Pain in Infants and Children.* Chapman & Hall, London.
10 Weinman J (1987) *An Outline of Psychology as Applied to Medicine.* (2nd edn) Wright, Bristol.
11 Price S (1990) Pain: Its experience, assessment and management in children. *Nurs Times.* **86** (9): 42–5.
12 Llewellyn N (1994) Pain assessment and the use of morphine analgesia in children. *Paediatr Nurs.* **6** (1): 25–30.
13 Beales JG (1986) Cognitive development and the experience of pain. *Nursing.* **11**: 408–10.
14 Zborowski M (1969) *People in Pain.* Jossey-Bass, San Francisco.
15 Ramsay J (1995) A genuine reflection of real needs: factors affecting pain assessment in children. *Child Health.* **3** (1): 20–4.

16   Levy D (1960) The infant's early memory of inoculation. *J Genet Psych.* **96** (3): 46.

17   Alex M and Ritchie JA (1992) School-aged children's interpretation of their experience with acute surgical pain. *Pediatr Nurs.* **7** (3): 171–88.

18   Eland J (1990) Pain in children. *Nurs Clin North Am.* **25** (4): 871–84.

19   Wong D and Baker C (1988) Pain in children: comparison of assessment scales. *Pediatr Nurs.* **14** (1): 9–17.

20   Baker C and Wong D (1987) QUESTT: a process of pain assessment in children. *Orthopaed Nurs.* **6** (1): 11–21.

21   Burr S (1987) Pain in childhood. *Nursing.* **24**: 890–4.

22   Ellis JA (1988) Using pain scales to prevent under-medication. *MCN.* **13**: 180–2.

23   Eland J (1985) The child who is hurting. *Semin Oncol Nurs.* **1**: 116–22.

24   Gadish HS, Gonzalez JL and Hayes JS (1988) Factors affecting nurses' decisions to administer pediatric pain medication post-operatively. *Pediatr Nurs.* **3** (6): 383–9.

25   Schofield P (1995) Using assessment tools to help patients in pain. *Profession Nurse.* **10** (11): 703–6.

26   May L (1992) Reducing pain and anxiety in children. *Nurs Standard.* **6** (44): 25–8.

27   McGrath PJ, Unrah AM and Finley GA (1995) Pain measurement in children. *Pain: Clin Updates.* **3** (2): 1–4.

28   Mather L and Mackie J (1983) The incidence of post-operative pain in children. *Pain.* **15**: 271–82.

29   Gildea JH and Quirk TR (1977) Assessing the pain experience in children. *Nurs Clin North Am.* **1**: 631–7.

30   Price PS (1992) Student nurses' assessment of children in pain. *J Adv Nurs.* **17**: 441–7.

31   Nethercott SG (1994) The assessment and management of post-operative pain in children by registered sick children's nurses: an exploratory study. *J Clin Nurs.* **3**: 109–14.

32   McCory LB (1991) A review of the second symposium of paediatric pain. *Pediatr Nurs.* **17** (4): 366–70.

33   Berker M and Hughes B (1990) Using a tool for pain assessment. *Nurs Times.* **86** (24): 50–2.

34   Royal College of Paediatrics and Child Health (1997) *Prevention and Control of Pain.* BMJ Publishing Group, London.

35   McGrath PJ, Ritchie JA and Unrah AM (1993) Paediatric pain. In: *Pain Management and Nursing Care* (eds D Carroll and D Bowsher). Butterworth-Heinemann, Oxford.

36   Ball AJ and Ferguson S (1996) Analgesia and analgesic drugs in paediatrics. *Br J Hosp Med.* **55** (9): 586–90.

37   Qureshi J and Buckingham S (1994) A pain assessment tool for all children. *Paediatr Nurs.* **6** (7): 11–13.

38   Melzack R (1987) The short-form McGill Pain Questionnaire. *Pain.* **30**: 191–7.

39   Jerrett M and Evans K (1986) Children's pain vocabulary. *J Adv Nurs.* **11**: 403–8.

40   Wilkie DJ, Savedra MC, Holzemer WL *et al.* (1990) Use of the McGill Pain Questionnaire to measure pain: a meta-analysis. *Nurs Res.* **39**: 36–41.

41   Varni JW, Thompson KL and Hanson V (1987) The Varni-Thompson Pediatric Pain Questionnaire 1: chronic musculoskeletal pain in juvenile rheumatoid arthritis. *Pain.* **28**: 27–38.

42 Beyer JE and Aradine CR (1986) Content validity of an instrument to measure young children's perceptions of their pain. *Pediatr Nurs.* **1**: 386–95.

43 Tyler DC, Douhit A-TJ and Chapman CR (1993) Towards a validation of pain measurement tools for children: a pilot study. *Pain.* **52**: 301–9.

44 Sellitz C, Wrightsman LS and Cook SW (1976) *Research Methods in Social Relations.* (3rd edn) Holt, Rinehart & Winston, New York.

45 McGuire DB (1984) The measurement of clinical pain. *Nurs Res.* **33** (3): 152–6.

46 Morse JM (1989) *Qualitative Nursing Research: A Contemporary Dialogue.* Sage, London.

47 Oppenheim AN (1984) *Questionnaire Design and Attitude Measurement.* Heinemann, London.

48 Meinhart NT and McCaffery M (1983) *Pain: a nursing approach to assessment and evaluation.* Appleton & Lange, East Norwalk, CT.

49 Gillies M (1995) In: *Child Health Care Nursing: concepts, theory and practice* (eds B Carter and A Dearmun). Blackwell Scientific, Oxford.

6 Pain assessment in the pre-verbal child

Introduction

Assessment of neonatal pain remains inconsistent.[1]

'The burden of proof should be shifted to those who maintain that infants do not feel pain.'[2]

Try to imagine yourself as a pre-verbal child. You speak a language that no-one understands and for which there are no interpreters. You are being assessed by people who have no recollection of their time as an infant and, therefore, cannot relate to your situation. You are constantly developing and gaining new skills and behaviours, which means that the methods you use to communicate pain as a premature neonate are different from those you use as a 10-month-old infant. These factors mean that assessing pain in the pre-verbal child is extremely difficult. This chapter will review the current thinking and highlight some of the pitfalls in the assessment of pain in the pre-verbal child.

Who is defined as a pre-verbal child?

The category of the pre-verbal child includes far more than infants and small children.

Children who are unable to use self-report pain assessment tools fit into the category of the pre-verbal child. The category of the pre-verbal child includes:

- children too young to communicate verbally or understand instructions
- the mentally handicapped child who may be 10 years old but may have the mind of a two year-old
- some physically handicapped children, particularly those who are blind or deaf

- children in the intensive care unit who may be intubated (and unable to vocalize) and paralysed (and unable to move)

- children whose consciousness is clouded as they recover from anaesthesia or following a head injury.

Consequences of unrelieved pain in pre-verbal children

The consequences of unrelieved pain are discussed in Chapter 1. Failure to relieve pain in neonates can cause other problems, for example:

- can affect the parent–infant bond due to the behavioural changes associated with pain[3]

- may result in an increased incidence of intraventricular haemorrhage.[4]

Problems with pre-verbal children and pain assessment

As adults we have virtually no recall of early life experiences. We cannot remember what caused us particular hurt and, more importantly, we cannot remember how we responded to that hurt.

As adults we have experienced a wide range of physical and emotional pain. Our previous experiences affect not only our response to painful stimuli but also our perception of those stimuli. For example, if we undergo surgery, we expect it to hurt. But:

- we can communicate that pain to others so that they can relieve the pain

- we have experience of pain and we can place this new pain in context

- we know from previous experience that the pain will eventually get better

- we know of people who have undergone similar operations or procedures and survived.

A 12 month-old child does not know any of this. As they are pre-verbal, these children cannot verbally communicate that they are in pain. Therefore any pain assessment must depend upon certain assumptions. These are discussed in the sections that follow.

What is painful to an adult is painful to an infant or child unless proven otherwise[5]

- This should alert the health care professional to look for features in the child's behaviour suggesting pain.

Different types of pain may elicit different responses

- Many assessments of the pain response have been developed from observations following a discrete noxious stimulus, for example, a needle stick or heel lance.

- The response seen does not necessarily translate to other types of pain, such as post-operative pain; different types of pain may elicit different responses.

Healthy pre-verbal children do not have the same pain response as children who are unwell

- Sick children, and particularly those with a mental handicap, have different pain responses from healthy children.

- Very little research has been done in trying to develop a pain assessment tool for the mentally handicapped child; this remains one of the most difficult areas of paediatric pain assessment.

Pain and the pre-verbal child

It is now agreed that small children, including neonates, are capable of experiencing pain. The evidence for this is based on both anatomical and physiological data.

Anatomical

- To experience pain from a noxious (tissue damaging) stimulus, there must be a pathway from the site of injury to the brain.

- The brain must be sufficiently developed to be able to perceive that noxious stimulus as being painful.

- From an early age, the fetus can experience pain.
- The newborn baby has the capability to feel pain.[3,6]

Physiological

- Studies have demonstrated that babies, both premature and term, are able to mount a stress response to a noxious stimulus and that either anaesthesia or the use of opioids can modify the response.[7,8]
- These studies demonstrate results very similar to those seen in adults.

Assessment techniques

If we accept that small children, including neonates, have the anatomical and physiological capacity to experience pain, it is essential that we have tools or techniques to detect that pain.

- The ideal method would be to get children to tell us whether they are in pain, how severe the pain is and whether the analgesia that we are giving is relieving the pain sufficiently.[10]
- Self-report methods are not available when dealing with pre-verbal children.
- Other pointers to distress and pain, such as physiological markers of stress and pain-associated behaviours, have to be used.

Before using an assessment tool in clinical practice, the tool must be tested to determine whether it achieves what you want.

- Does the tool discriminate between pain and other causes of distress (validity)?
  - there are many reasons why a baby might cry, such as hunger, anxiety, cold, unhappiness and pain
  - if you are using a child's cry as a marker of pain, your tool must be able to separate pain cries from all other cries.

- Will your tool give the same results when used by two different people at the same time or by you at different times (reliability)?
  - establishing reliability can be difficult
  - a child's pain may fluctuate, if two different results are obtained, say 15 minutes apart, this may be due to either a genuine change in the child's pain or two different interpretations of the same level of pain.

(The validity and reliability of pain assessment tools is discussed in Chapter 5.)

For a pain tool to be useful it must be:

- able to detect the presence of pain and discriminate pain from other causes of distress

- able to assess the severity of the pain
  - pain is a continuum rather than a discrete entity, therefore, a tool must be able to grade the severity of the pain

- able to determine the effectiveness of interventions
  - are your analgesic interventions relieving the pain? If pain is not relieved by treatment several questions need to be asked:
    - (i)   is an appropriate type and amount of analgesic prescribed?
    - (ii) is the analgesic being administered regularly?
    - (iii) is the pain due to other reasons? For example, a child who has had a laparotomy may have pain from the incision but also from a full bladder. The first requires more analgesia, the second may require urinary catheterization

- simple to use
  - this is essential. Highly complex and detailed tools that require detailed explanation are fine for research purposes but are of little use on busy wards. A simple tool assessing a limited number of variables (less than 10) is much more likely to be adopted and used successfully on a busy ward

- appropriate for the child's cognitive development
  - premature infants show different behaviour patterns from small children.[11,12] A useful test in one age group need not necessarily be so in another.

Children's cognitive development and their perception of pain is discussed in Chapter 2. Some general guidelines for managing pain in children can be found in Chapter 5.

Behavioural methods of assessing pain in the pre-verbal child

In recent years, patterns of behaviour in the neonate have been increasingly studied. The behaviours examined have been:[13]

- facial expression
- body/limb movements
- crying.

Before discussing these aspects of behaviour it must be emphasized that there are major developmental changes in behaviour from a premature neonate to a pre-verbal two year-old.[14]

Facial expression

'Whilst thus screaming their eyes are firmly closed, so that the skin round them is wrinkled, and the forehead contracted into a frown. The mouth is widely opened with the lips retracted in a peculiar manner, which causes it to assume a squarish form; the gums or teeth being more or less exposed. The breath is inhaled almost spasmodically.'[15]

Several observers have developed so-called facial coding systems with a view to aiding the classification of certain facial expressions.

- Craig developed a tool solely based on facial expressions and devised the neonatal facial acting coding system (NFCS).[16]
- This was then refined and the activities seen in response to pain were described as *pain expression*. These are:
  - eye squeeze
  - brow contraction
  - nasolabial furrow
  - taut tongue
  - open mouth.
- These facial expressions seem to apply to all babies in the premature to four month-old group.[17]
- The facial expressions vary with the initial sleep/awake state of the baby.

- The presence of a taut tongue or vertical mouth stretch (squarish mouth) showed the greatest change in the awake baby to the heel lance but showed the least changes in the sleeping state.

- The sleep/awake state of the baby should, therefore, be taken into account.

- Premature babies produce the same facial features as older babies but do so less vigorously.

- This was particularly evident with the more sick premature baby. There was a trend of decreasing change in facial expression with increasing ill-health.[17,19]

- The maximally discriminative facial movement coding system (MAX) has been shown to be able to separate a physical distress facial expression from that of anger.[20]

Body/limb movement

The evidence suggests that body movement in response to a painful stimulus can be used to assess pain in the pre-verbal child. Lack of response, however, does not indicate a lack of pain perception; it may indicate a greater intensity of pain.

- Early examination of the response to a pinprick in neonates suggested that the response was a diffuse, reflex response.

- More detailed examination finds that, in addition to the reflex withdrawal response, there is often a contralateral limb response trying to remove the noxious stimulus, suggesting that the response is more than purely reflex.

- Body and limb movements during acute insults have been examined. With an injection, there is an immediate rigid phase rapidly followed by thrashing of the limbs.[21]

- A similar picture of torso squirming and limb movements is seen immediately after surgery if analgesia has been inadequate.

- This behaviour responds to analgesia.

- If the child is followed into the later post-operative period, the child learns that moving is painful, whether it be an abdominal wound or a broken wrist.

- It must be emphasized that absence of movement does not mean absence of pain and may mean more pain rather than less.

- In a detailed study of three post-operative neonates following major surgery one infant received one tenth the analgesia of the other two. This infant, in addition to showing acute and subacute distress, also showed *jerky startles.*[16]

- These jerky startles are well recognized in neonates confronted with repetitive disturbing stimuli, where the infant goes into a deep sleep, has tense and flexed limbs and jerky startles.[16]

- This state is often mistaken for too much analgesia, when in fact the infant requires more analgesia not less.[16]

- The richness and vigour of an infant's response to pain was often relied upon by nurses when making an assessment of pain intensity.[22]

- Significantly higher pain scores were allocated to the full-term babies than to pre-term infants.

- This suggests that the noisier, more reactive babies received more recognition and attention than the quieter, less responsive infants.

- This has serious implications for the pre-term infant in the neonatal intensive care unit, as lack of response to a situation may signify a lack of capability, rather than a lack of pain perception.

Crying

Research indicates that there is a typical cry in response to a painful stimulus. This is not considered a reliable indicator on its own and should be used in conjunction with other indicators of pain.

Lack of response (crying) does not indicate a lack of pain.

- Early work suggests that infant crying in response to pain or pain-induced vocalization (PIV) is very promising.[23]

- Animal and human studies show that PIV has an immediate and potent effect on parental behaviour.[23]

- Mothers are able to distinguish between PIV and other types of cry.[23]

- Studies on animals have shown that PIV is a high level (thalamic) response and that PIV is the only animal pain response that is blocked by opioids at doses used to treat human pain, suggesting that PIV may be specific for pain.[23]

- In healthy term infants, cry type alone is not reliable enough to be useful in pain assessment.

- Type of cry is most useful when combined with facial expression as a composite assessment tool.

- There is still too much cry variation between babies in their response to acute pain to make it a reliable tool on its own.

- Some of this variability may be inherent in the premature baby's inability to modulate its cries.[24]

- As many as 50% of pre-term neonates do not cry after a painful event; lack of response may not mean lack of perception.[25]

Physiological methods of assessing pain in the pre-verbal child

Physiological methods are a useful tool for assessing pain in the pre-verbal child.

If pain persists over a period of time there is less of an increase in the sympathetic responses. This phenomenon is known as adaptation.[26]

- Currently a specific variable for pain does not exist.

- Most research has centred around finding variables that change with pain, as well as other forms of stress, and seeing whether a combination of these variables would produce patterns of responses that were more specific for pain than the individual variables themselves.

- Physiological variables largely measure stress. Pain is only one of many causes of stress so that unless the only cause of the child's stress is pain these variables are not specific to pain.

- Physiological variables have certain potential advantages over other forms of pain assessment:
    - they do not require the child's co-operation and are objective
    - can be used in situations where other forms of assessment would be impossible, such as in the intensive care unit
    - physiological variables are objective measurements and usually produce data of interval or ratio quality, thereby allowing more powerful analysis of the data.

- These may be used inappropriately by nurses at times when adaptation to pain could have been expected to have occurred.[27]
- They should be used in conjunction with other indicators of pain.
- There are three types of physiological indicators used to assess pain in the pre-verbal child:
    - cardiovascular variables
    - respiratory variables
    - metabolic and endocrine variables.

Cardiovascular variables

- Includes heart rate, blood pressure, skin galvanic response and palmar sweating.
- It is important to remember that there are many causes of alterations in these variables. For example, an increased heart rate may be due to pain, but also shock, such as hypovolaemia or sepsis.
- If several variables are examined together, such as heart rate and blood pressure, a more specific and useful picture appears.

Respiratory variables

- Includes respiratory rate, transcutaneous oxygen tension and pulse oximetry.[29]
- It is common to find children, following thoracic or abdominal surgery, who have a rapid respiratory rate, with shallow respirations and a decreased oxygen saturation.
- This pattern is often seen if the child is in pain as shallow breathing is less painful than deeper breathing.
- If these children are given analgesia their respiratory rate decreases, the breathing gets deeper and the oxygen saturation rises.[30]

Metabolic and endocrine variables

- Includes the stress hormones, such as adrenaline, noradrenaline and cortisol, metabolic products, such as free fatty acids, glucose and markers of protein breakdown.[3,6,29-31]

Generally several variables, including behavioural variables, used in combination are more effective than variables used in isolation. To optimize the usefulness and specificity of physiological variables in the assessment of pain, proper clinical assessment of the child is essential to exclude other causes of stress.

Pain assessment tools for the pre-verbal child

Box 6.1 provides details of the tools available for use in neonates. The parameters used to assess pain are listed and details of research studies given.

Box 6.2 provides details of the pain assessment tools available for use in infants and young children.

Further research is needed in this area to enable health care professionals to assess pain in the pre-verbal child effectively. It would appear that a combination of parameters provides the best measure of a pre-verbal child's pain intensity.

When using a pain assessment tool it is important to record the pain score obtained on a flow chart designed specifically for the purpose. This ensures continuity of care and helps communication between members of the multidisciplinary team.

Role of the parents

- Parents may notice subtle changes in their baby that may escape the attentions of the nurse.

- Parents' involvement should not be taken for granted.

- Nurses often think parents are the best people to assess their child's pain but parents may be stressed and may have little experience of seeing their child in pain.[48]

- Parents often expect the nurse to know when their child is in pain.[48]

Summary

- If optimal pain control is to be achieved in the pre-verbal child it is vital that we are able to assess that child's pain and monitor the effectiveness of analgesia upon that pain.

Box 6.1   Assessment tools for neonates

Assessment tool	Parameters	Findings
CRIES[32]	*Crying* (none, high pitched, inconsolable) *O₂ requirement* (none, <30%, >30%) *Increased vital signs* (HR and or BP as pre-op, <30% increase, >30% increase) *Facial expression* (none, grimace, grunt) *Sleepless* (no, wakes, always awake)	• good inter-observer validity • validated in neonates up to 72 h after surgery
Neonatal infant pain scale (NIPS)[33]	• facial expression • cry • breathing patterns • arms • legs • state of arousal Zero score for intubated patients	• used in premature and term neonates • good validity and reliability • only validated for heel pricks, not after major surgery
Rushforth[34,35]	• brow bulge • eye squeeze • nasolabial furrow • open mouth • crying	• good inter-observer agreement after heel pricks • infant arousal state did not affect pain scores • could not discern between lignocaine and placebo

Box 6.1   Continued

Assessment tool	Parameters	Findings
Ramenghi and Haouari[36-38]	• facial (brow bulge, eye squeeze, nasolabial furrow, open mouth) – present or absent • cry (total cry time, and % >5 min) • heart rate • O_2 saturation	• useful for showing the benefits of sucrose or sweetener against pain from heel pricks • most sensitive indicator was cry • combined behavioural and physiological score

Box 6.2   Pain assessment tools for infants and young children

Assessment tool	Parameters	Findings
CHEOPS[39-41]	• cry • facial expression • verbal • torso • touch • legs	• validated in 1–5 year-olds after surgery • good inter-observer reliability • effective in the immediate post-operative period • not valid after this period because children learn to keep still • now modified (mCHEOPS) to make assessment simpler
Toddler pre-school post-operative pain scale (TPPPS)[42]	• vocal expression • facial expression • bodily expression	• simple to perform, either +(=)1 or –(=)0 • good inter-rater reliability • only validated for immediate post-operative period
Nursing assessment of pain intensity (NAPI)[43,44]	• verbal/vocal • body movement • facial • touching	• adapted from CHEOPS score • good reliability
Pain/discomfort score[45]	• blood pressure • crying • movement • agitation • posture • complains of pain	• investigated children after orchidopexy • found no difference between ileoinguinal and caudal nerve blocks

Box 6.2 Continued

Assessment tool	Parameters	Findings
Paediatric objective pain score[46]	• as for the pain/discomfort tool but without *complains of pain*	• used successfully in children two months to 10 years
Post-operative pain score[47]	• sleep during preceding hour • facial expression • quality of cry • spontaneous movement • spontaneous excitability • flexion of fingers/toes • sucking • global evaluation of tone • consolability • sociability	• used in the comparison of two groups of infants in the two hours following minor surgery • one group received intra-operative fentanyl; the other group received no opioids • observers rated 54% of the fentanyl group to have adequate analgesia • only 18% of placebo group were observed to have adequate analgesia

- In the pre-verbal child we are limited to behavioural and physiological variables.

- There is currently no behavioural or physiological variable or score that is specific for pain.

- We must therefore rely upon the assumption that if children have had something potentially painful done to them they will feel pain.

- If a child shows behaviours or physiological changes suggestive of stress, in the presence of having something potentially painful done, it is likely that the stress response is due to pain.

- Assuming that what would hurt us, as adults, would probably hurt a child, the detection of pain in the pre-verbal child becomes simpler.

- There are a number of pain assessment tools available that combine physiological and behavioural variables in order to establish the intensity of a pre-verbal child's pain.

References

1   Carlson KL, Clement BA and Nash P (1996) Neonatal pain: from concept to research questions and a role for the advanced practice nurse. *J Perinatal Neonatal Nurs.* **10** (1): 64–71.
2   Owens ME (1984) Pain in infancy: Conceptual and methodological issues. *Pain.* **20**: 213–30.
3   Anand KJS and Hickey PR (1987) Pain and its effects in the human neonate and fetus. *N Engl J Med.* **317**: 1321–9.
4   Shapiro CR (1993) Nurses judgement of pain in term and pre-term newborns. *J Obstet Gynecol Neonatal Nurses.* **22** (1): 41–7.
5   Franck LS (1989) Pain in the non-verbal patient: advocating for the critically ill neonate. *Paediatr Nurs.* **15**: 65–8.
6   Anand KJS and Carr DB (1989) The neuroanatomy, neurophysiology, and neuro-chemistry of pain, stress, and analgesia in newborns and children. *Pediatr Clin North Am.* **36**: 795–822.
7   Anand KJS, Sippell WG and Aynsley-Green A (1987) Randomised trial of fentanyl anaesthesia in preterm babies undergoing surgery: effects on the stress response. *Lancet.* **1**: 243–8.
8   Anand KJS and Aynsley-Green A (1988) Does the newborn infant require potent anesthesia during surgery? Answers from a randomized trial of halothane anesthesia. In: *Proceedings of the Vth World Congress on Pain* (eds R Dubner, GK Gebhart and MR Bond). Elsevier Science Publishers, Amsterdam.
9   Richmond CE, Bromley LA and Woolf CJ (1993) Preoperative morphine pre-empts postoperative pain. *Lancet.* **342**: 73–5.
10   Porter F in Phillips P (1995) Neonatal pain management: a call to action. *Paediatr Nurs.* **21**: 195–9.

11 Johnston CC, Stevens B, Craig KD et al. (1993) Development changes in premature, full term, two and four month old infants. *Pain.* **52**: 201–8.

12 Stevens B and Johnston C (1992) Assessment and management of pain in infants. *Can Nurse.* **Aug**: 31–4.

13 Hodgkinson K, Bear M, Thorn J et al. (1994) Measuring pain in neonates: Evaluating an instrument and developing a common language. *Aust J Adv Nurs.* **12** (1): 17–22.

14 McGraw MB (1941) Neural maturation as exemplified in the changing reactions of the infant to pin prick. *Child Dev.* **12**: 31–42.

15 Darwin C (first published 1872), (1965) Special expressions of man: suffering and weeping. In: *The Expression of the Emotions in Man and Animals.* University of Chicago Press, Chicago, p. 147.

16 Grunau RVE and Craig KD (1987) Pain expression in neonates: facial action and cry. *Pain.* **28**: 395–410.

17 Johnston CC and Strada ME (1986) Acute pain response in infants: a multi-dimensional description. *Pain.* **24**: 373–82.

18 Grunau RVE, Johnston CC and Craig KD (1990) Neonatal facial and cry responses to invasive and non-invasive procedures. *Pain.* **42**: 295–305.

19 Stevens BJ, Johnston CC and Horton L (1994) Factors that influence the behavioral responses of premature infants. *Pain.* **59**: 101–9.

20 Izard CE, Hembree EA, Dougherty LM and Spizzirri CC (1983) Changes in facial expression of 2- to 19-month old infants following acute pain. *Dev Psych.* **19**: 418–26.

21 Cote JJ, Morse JM and James SG (1991) The pain response of the postoperative newborn. *J Adv Nurs.* **16**: 378–87.

22 Shapiro CR (1993) Nurses judgements of pain in term and preterm newborns. *J Obstet Gynecol Neonatal Nurses.* **22** (1): 41–7.

23 Levine JD and Gordon NC (1982) Pain in prelingual children and its evaluation by pain-induced vocalization. *Pain.* **14**: 85–93.

24 Thodén C-J, Järvenpää A-L and Michelsson K (1985) Sound spectrographic cry analysis of pain cry in prematures. In: *Infant Crying: Theoretical and Research Perspectives* (eds BM Lester and CFZ Boukydis). Plenum Press, New York.

25 Stevens BJ and Johnston CC (1994) Physiological responses of premature infants to painful stimulus. *Nurs Res.* **43**: 226–31.

26 Gildea JH, Quirk JH and Quirk TH (1977) Assessing the pain experience in children. *Nurs Clin North Am.* **1**: 631–7.

27 Price PS (1992) Student nurses' assessment of children in pain. *J Adv Nurs.* **17**: 441–7.

28 Nethercott SG (1994) The assessment and management of post-operative pain in children by registered sick children's nurses: an exploratory study. *J Clin Nurs.* **3**: 109–14.

29 Geisen G, Frederiksen PS, Hertel J et al. (1985) Catecholamine response to chest physiotherapy and endotracheal suctioning in preterm infants. *Acta Paediatr Scand.* **74**: 525–9.

30 Bara H, Maekawa N, Tanaka O et al. (1984) Plasma cortisol levels in paediatric anaesthesia. *Can Anaesth Soc J.* **31**: 24–7.

31 Srinivasan G, Jain R, Pildes RS et al. (1986) Glucose homeostasis during anesthesia and surgery in infants. *J Pediatr Surg.* **21**: 718–21.

32   Krechel SW and Bildner J (1995) CRIES A new neonatal postoperative pain measurement score. Initial testing of validity and reliability. *Paediatr Anaesth.* **5**: 53–61.

33   Lawrence J, Alcock D, McGrath P *et al.* (1993) The development of a tool to assess neonatal pain. *Neonatal Network.* **12**: 59–65.

34   Rushforth JA and Levene MI (1994) Behavioural response to pain in healthy neonates. *Arch Dis Child.* **70**: F174–6.

35   Rushforth JA, Griffiths GC, Thorpe H *et al.* (1995) Can topical lignocaine reduce behavioural response to heel prick. *Arch Dis Child.* **72**: F49–51.

36   Ramenghi LA, Griffiths GC, Wood CM *et al.* (1996) Effect of non-sucrose sweet tasting solution on neonatal heel prick responses. *Arch Dis Child.* **74**: F129–31.

37   Haouari N, Wood C, Griffiths GC *et al.* (1995) The analgesic effect of sucrose in full term infants: a randomised controlled trial. *BMJ.* **310**: 1498–500.

38   Ramenghi LA, Wood CM, Griffiths GC *et al.* (1996) Reduction of pain response in premature infants using intra-oral sucrose. *Arch Dis Child.* **74**: F126–28.

39   McGrath PJ, Johnson G, Goodman JT *et al.* (1985) CHEOPS: A behavioral scale for rating postoperative pain in children. In: *Advances in Pain Research and Therapy* (ed. HL Fields). Raven Press, New York, pp. 395–402.

40   Beyer JE, McGrath PJ and Berde CB (1990) Discordance between self-report and behavioural pain measures in children aged 3–7 years after surgery. *J Pain Symptom Manage.* **5**: 350–6.

41   Splinter WM, Semelhago LC and Chou S (1994) The reliability and validity of a modified CHEOPS pain score. *Anesth Analg.* **78**: S413.

42   Tarbell SE, Cohen IT and Marsh JL (1992) The Toddler-Preschooler Postoperative Pain Scale: an observational scale for measuring postoperative pain in children aged 1-5. Preliminary report. *Pain.* **50**: 273–80.

43   Stevens B (1990) Development and testing of a pediatric pain management sheet. *Pediatr Nurs.* **16**: 543–8.

44   Joyce BA, Schade JG, Keck JF *et al.* (1994) Reliability and validity of preverbal pain assessment tools. *Iss Comprehensive Nurs.* **17**: 121–35.

45   Barrier G, Attia J, Mayer MN *et al.* (1989) Measurement of postoperative pain and narcotic administration in infants using a new clinical scoring system. *Intensive Care Med.* **15**: S37–9.

46   Hannallah RS, Broadman LM, Belman AS *et al.* (1987) Comparison of caudal and ileo-inguinal/ilio-hypogastric nerve blocks for control of post orchidopexy pain in pediatric ambulatory surgery. *Anaesth.* **66**: 832–4.

47   Conroy JM, Otherson HB, Dorman BH *et al.* (1993) A comparison of wound instillation and caudal block for analgesia following pediatric inguinal herniorrhaphy. *J Pediatr Surg.* **28**: 565–7.

48   Eland J (1985) The child who is hurting. *Semin Oncol Nurs.* **1**: 116–22.

7 Non-drug methods of pain control

Introduction

> We have learnt as a result of literally hundreds of experiments, that there is a limit to the effectiveness of any given therapy; but happily the effects of two or more therapies given in conjunction are cumulative.[1]

This chapter will provide an overview of some of the most commonly used non-drug methods available to aid the relief of pain in children. It is important for health care professionals to remember that, with certain exceptions such as the use of cold, non-drug methods do not relieve the child's pain – they simply dull their perception of the pain. The pain is still there but the intensity of pain perception is decreased. Over the last few years non-drug methods have become more widely used in children although many of the methods are still under-researched. The usefulness of non-drug methods will be discussed and several of the non-drug methods will be described.

Usefulness of non-drug methods

> Non-drug methods of pain control are probably most effective as coping strategies, not for actual reduction of the intensity of pain. Although there are exceptions to this statement, such as the use of cold, the most likely outcome of techniques such as relaxation and distraction is that pain will be more tolerable, not necessarily less severe in intensity.[2]

- Many non-drug techniques can be taught or facilitated by nurses so that children and their families can take over this part of their pain management giving the child and family some control over the management of their pain.[3]

- Non-drug methods of pain control may be overused or even abused with certain children or in some circumstances. Children who are co-operative and adept at techniques such as distraction may actually suffer in silence and not be provided with appropriate analgesia or local anaesthesia.[2]

- Adequate pharmacological control must be used as and when necessary; additional methods of reducing pain and anxiety will help the child relax and cope better with pain and distress.[4]

Non-drug methods can be divided into two groups:

- counterirritation
- psychological methods.

Examples of each type can be seen in Box 7.1. Chapter 8 provides more detailed discussion of some of the psychological methods of pain relief. Several of the non-drug methods will now be discussed.

Sometimes non-drug methods alone will be adequate. Generally, however, they are used in conjunction with drug and other non-drug methods. Not all patients will find them beneficial.[5]

Box 7.1 Examples of counterirritation and psychological methods of pain relief[5]

Counterirritation	Psychological methods
Heat	Distraction
Cold	Imagery
Chemicals	Relaxation
Massage	Music therapy
Transcutaneous electrical nerve stimulation	Biofeedback
Acupuncture	Hypnosis
Vibration	Cognitive-behavioural therapy

Distraction

Distraction appears best in helping the child to deal with relatively short duration pain such as procedural pain.[3]

- Makes pain more tolerable or bearable by putting pain at the periphery of awareness.[6]
- Attention is focused on the distracter rather than the pain.[3]

- Although it does not reduce the intensity of pain it is often an effective coping strategy for pre-school and older children.

- To determine an effective distraction strategy the nurse involves the child and parents in identifying what is particularly interesting to the child.[2]

The characteristics of effective distraction strategies for brief episodes of pain are:[2]

- interesting to the child

- consistent with the child's energy level and ability to concentrate

- if music or poetry, rhythm is included and emphasized

- stimulates the major sensory modalities:
  - hearing
  - vision
  - touch
  - movement

- capable of providing a change in stimuli when the pain changes, for example, increasing stimuli as pain increases.

Box 7.2 suggests ways of using distraction with children. Care needs to be taken to choose a strategy appropriate to the child's age, and his or her likes and dislikes.

Box 7.2   Distraction strategies for use with children[2,4,7]

- Holding a familiar object (comforter), such as a pillow or cuddly toy
- Singing; concentrating on nice things; telling jokes; games and puzzles
- Going on imaginary journeys
- Blowing air bubbles
- Blowing an imaginary feather off the doctor's nose
- Reading pop-up books
- Playing with a kaleidoscope or 3D viewer
- Breathing out
- Looking in a mirror to see the view through a nearby window
- Watching television or a video; playing interactive computer games
- Listening through headphones to stories or music

Parents can help with a number of these activities but will need guidance from health care professionals as to how they can help their child.

Children who use distraction techniques may look as if they are not in pain; health care professionals need to remember that distraction does not take away the pain.

Relaxation

Relaxation does not usually reduce the intensity of pain but it does reduce the distress associated with pain.[2]

Since a patient cannot be relaxed and anxious simultaneously, pain tolerance should be increased if the patient is relaxed.[8]

- An effective coping strategy for procedural, chronic or on-going pain.[2]

- For pain that lasts most of the day a relaxation technique may be performed several times a day.[2]

- Presence of a parent is useful in helping to reduce distress associated with pain for all age groups.[2]

- A young child can be made to relax simply by holding him or her in a comfortable well-supported position or rocking in a wide rhythmical arc in a rocking chair.

- Infants often display jerky movements in response to pain; rocking and comforting the baby appears to relieve this.[9]

- With a toddler or older child, blowing bubbles can be distracting and can eventually evolve into a type of relaxation technique in the form of rhythmical breathing without the bubbles.

- Ideally taught prior to painful procedures.

- May be used to reduce distress before and during a painful procedure.

Transcutaneous electrical nerve stimulation (TENS)

Useful in localized pain – thought to increase endorphin levels and act as a counterirritant.[10]

- Little research in its use in paediatrics.[11]
- Should be used in combination with other treatment methods.[11]
- TENS aims to relieve pain and is non-invasive and safe.[11]
- The TENS device delivers controlled low voltage electricity to the body via electrodes.[11]
- TENS recipients often describe a sensation of tingling when the device is working.[7]
- Useful for both acute and chronic pain.[12]
- Is non-invasive and, therefore, the development of this method for paediatric use should be encouraged.

Imagery

The use of imagination to modify the response to pain.[13]

Provides relief through distraction, relaxation and producing an image of pain.[7]

- Involves using sensory images that modify the pain to make it more bearable or to substitute a pleasant image in place of pain.[10]
- Can be used in a guided way so that the child imagines something about his or her pain that will help to reduce it – for example, children who have pain can picture the pain flowing out of their bodies.[3]

Massage

The systematic manual manipulation of the soft tissues of the body to produce relaxation of the muscles.[14]

- Promotes circulation of the blood, relief from pain, restoration of meta-bolic balance as well as other physical and emotional benefits.[14]
- An ancient method of maintaining and improving health.[10]
- Children should be involved in the decision-making process and where appropriate give their permission.[3]

Touch

Many children, despite being cared for in a loving hospital environ-ment, are deprived of affective and therapeutic touch – even though they are at risk from a high level of instrumental touch.[3]

- Touch is a two-way process involving sensation and cognition.[3]
- The need to be touched is present at birth and is a continuing and developing need.[3]
- Provides one of the strongest means of communicating caring and empathy.[3]
- The average number of touches in a neonatal unit was five touches per 24 hours.[15]
- Staff other than nurses rarely touch the patients except to do a physical examination, and nurses touched the children most often when they were performing procedures.[16]

Aromatherapy

An holistic form of healing that uses essential oils extracted from aromatic plants.[17]

- Increasingly used as a means of reducing stress, relaxing, treating symptoms and providing relief from pain.[17]
- Promotes healing on different levels – physical, emotional and mental.[17]
- Should only be practised by a trained practitioner.[17]

Acupuncture

A system of ancient medicine, healing and Eastern philosophy originating in China.[18]

- The Chinese explanation of how acupuncture works is based on the idea that life force flows round certain lines on the body known as *meridians*.[19]
- Needling points on these lines is thought to correct an abnormal flow of life forces.[20]
- Another explanation is that acupuncture stimulates the production of natural endorphins.[19]
- It is particularly helpful in treating chronic pain; not effective in treating advanced cancer pain.[12]

Hypnosis

Defined as focused attention, an altered state of consciousness or a trance, often accompanied by relaxation.[21]

- Found to be of value in the care and management of children with both acute and chronic pain.[3]
- Does not actually take away the pain but decreases/removes the child's perception of it.[3]

Non-drug methods for infants

The administration of a sucrose solution to pre-term infants prior to heel lance procedures appears to decrease the pain/distress experienced by infants.[22]

Several studies have demonstrated the analgesic effects of non-nutritive sucking using sweet-tasting solutions in full and pre-term babies.[22–24]

- When different concentrations of sucrose solution were used a reduction in crying time was found with increasing concentrations of sucrose.[23]

- Sucrose alone was found to have an analgesic effect in pre-term infants which is enhanced by simulated rocking.[24]

- Further studies are required in this area.

> Quieting techniques that can be used with infants include holding and rocking, swaddling/nesting, assisting with hand-to-mouth contact and soothing sounds. These measures should be individualized according to the infant's likes and dislikes.

Training needs

Many of the non-drug methods described in this chapter can be used by health care professionals with very little training; others such as aromatherapy and hypnosis require a recognized qualification. It is important that health care professionals do not implement methods of which they have little or no knowledge. Utilizing the skills of the multi-disciplinary team is important; play therapists and clinical psychologists have a vital role in implementing non-drug methods.

Over the past five years the use of non-drug methods in paediatric pain management has increased. Further research is needed in some areas to evaluate the effectiveness of the methods. The implementation of non-drug methods in clinical practice, after appropriate training, should be encouraged.

Summary

- There are a number of non-drug methods of pain relief.

- These should be used in conjunction with analgesic drugs in order to control pain; many of the non-drug methods make the pain more tolerable rather than decreasing the intensity of the pain.

- Non-drug methods can be divided into counterirritation and psychological methods.

- Many of the non-drug methods need further research to validate their use with children.

- Many of the non-drug methods can be taught or facilitated by nurses.

- This means that children and families can take over part of their pain management.

- Some methods require training before health professionals implement them.

- The use of the multi-disciplinary team – particularly play therapists and clinical psychologists – is vital in the implementation of non-drug methods.

- The implementation of non-drug methods should be encouraged.

References

1   Melzack R and Whall PD (1982) *The Challenge of Pain*. Penguin Books, London.
2   McCaffery M and Wong D (1993) Nursing interventions for pain control in children. In: *Pain in Infants, Children and Adolescents* (eds NL Schechter, CB Berde and M Yaster). Williams & Wilkins, Baltimore, pp. 295–316.
3   Carter B (1994) *Child and Infant Pain: Principles of Nursing Care and Management*. Chapman & Hall, London.
4   May L (1992) Reducing pain and anxiety in children. *Nurs Standard*. **6** (4): 25–8.
5   Twycross RG (1994) *Pain Relief in Advanced Cancer*. Churchill Livingstone, London.
6   McCaffery M (1990) Nursing approaches to nonpharmacological pain control. *Int J Nurs Stud*. **27** (1): 1–5.
7   Royal College of Paediatrics and Child Health (1997) *Prevention and Control of Pain in Children*. BMJ Publishing Group, London.
8   Weisenberg M (1980) Understanding pain phenomenon. Cited in Carter B (1994) *Child and Infant Pain: Principles of Nursing Care and Management*. Chapman & Hall, London.
9   Roop Moyer SM and Howe CJ (1991) Pediatric pain intervention in the PACU. *Crit Care Nurs Clin North Am*. **3** (1): 49–57.
10   McCaffery M and Beebe AB (1989) *Pain: Clinical Manual for Nursing Practice*. CV Mosby, St Louis.
11   Eland J (1993) The use of TENS with children. In: *Pain in Infants, Children and Adolescents* (eds NL Schechter, CB Berde and M Yaster). Williams & Wilkins, Baltimore, pp. 331–9.
12   Sofaer B (1992) *Pain: A Handbook for Nurses*. (2nd edn) Chapman & Hall, London.
13   Doody SB, Smith C and Webb J (1991) Non-pharmacological interventions for pain management. *Crit Care Nurs Clin North Am*. **3** (1): 69–75.
14   Beck M (1988) *The Theory and Practice of Therapeutic Massage*. Milady, New York.
15   Blackburn S and Bernard KE (1985) Cited in Carter B (1994) *Child and Infant Pain: Principles of Nursing Care and Management*. Chapman & Hall, London.
16   Mitchell P (1985) Critically ill children: the importance of touch in a high technological environment. *Nurs Admin Quarter*. **9** (4): 38–46.
17   Carter B (1995) Complementary therapies and the management of chronic pain. *Paediatr Nurs*. **7** (3): 18–22.

18 Yee JD, Lin Y-C and Aubuchon PA (1993) Acupuncture. In: *Pain in Infants, Children and Adolescents* (eds NL Schechter, CB Berde and M Yaster). Williams & Wilkins, Baltimore, pp. 341–8.

19 Mayer DJ, Price DD and Raffii A (1976) Antagonism and acupuncture analgesia in man by the narcotic antagonist naloxone. *Brain Res.* **121**: 368–77.

20 Mann F (1971) Cited in Sofaer B (1992) *Pain: A Handbook for Nurses.* (2nd edn) Chapman & Hall, London.

21 Valente SM (1991) Using hypnosis with children for pain management. *Oncol Nurs Forum.* **18** (4): 699–704.

22 Buclei HU, Moset T, Siebenthal KV *et al.* (1995) Sucrose reduces pain reaction to heel lancing in pre-term infants: a placebo-controlled randomised and masked study. *Pediatr Res.* **38** (3): 332–5.

23 Haouari N, Wood C, Griffiths GC *et al.* (1995) The analgesic effect of sucrose in full term infants: a randomised controlled trial. *BMJ.* **310**: 1498–500.

24 Johnston CC, Stevens BJ and Stremler R (1996) *Sucrose, but not simulated rocking, decreases pain response in preterm infants.* Paper presented at the VIIIth World Congress on Pain, Vancouver, Canada.

Further reading

Carter B (1994) *Child and Infant Pain: Principles of Nursing Care and Management.* Chapman & Hall, London, pp. 90–104.

Eland J (1989) The effectiveness of transcutaneous electrical nerve stimulation (TENS) with children experiencing cancer pain. In: *Management of Pain, Fatigue and Nausea* (eds SG Funk *et al.*). Macmillan, London, pp. 87–100.

Fowler-Kerry S and Ramsay-Lander J (1990) Utilizing cognitive strategies to relieve pain in young children. In: *Advances in Pain Research Therapy Vol. 15* (eds DC Tyler and EJ Krane). Raven Press, New York, pp. 247–53.

Hilgard ER and Hilgard JR (1983) *Hypnosis in the Relief of Pain.* (2nd edn) William Kaufman, Los Altos.

Hilgard JR and LeBaron S (1984) *Hypnotherapy of Pain in Children with Cancer.* William Kaufman, Los Altos.

McCaffery M and Beebe AB (1989) *Pain: Clinical Manual for Nursing Practice.* CV Mosby, St Louis, pp. 142–227.

Ryan EA (1989) The effect of musical distraction of pain, fatigue and nausea. In: *Management of Pain, Fatigue and Nausea* (eds SG Funk *et al.*). Macmillan, London, pp. 101–10.

Schechter NL, Berde CB and Yaster M (eds) (1993) *Pain in Infants, Children and Adolescents.* Williams & Wilkins, Baltimore, pp. 295–348.

Vessey JA, Carlson KL and McGill J (1994) Use of distraction with children during an acute painful experience. *Nurs Res.* **43** (6): 369–72.

8 The role of the clinical psychologist in paediatric pain management

Introduction

Research literature and reviews have shown that the psychological approaches to pain management are effective.[1,2]

The non-drug treatment of both acute and chronic pain in paediatrics has increasingly been the focus of applied psychology and psychophysiology. It is necessary to look at the problem of paediatric pain and its management by firstly examining the influences on the child and within the child, and then proceeding to the interface of the child–professional system. The manner in which health care professionals understand pain is not limited to academic discussions of the neurones, the transmission of pain impulses, and the physiological processes, nor to the subjective experiential pain. Professional understanding of pain needs to link these, and other aspects, in a multi-faceted way. Perhaps more importantly it needs to underpin and guide our practice and treatment of children in hospital. Only once there has been an agreed focus and interdisciplinary plan can the applications and techniques be implemented. It is the aim of this chapter to highlight this process. Chapter 7 provided an overview of non-drug methods of pain relief. This chapter will look at the role of the clinical psychologist (paediatric clinical psychology is still a fairly new discipline) and examine the psychological methods of pain relief in more detail.

The role of the clinical psychologist

To use psychological methods of pain control it is important to involve a paediatric clinical psychologist. Types of services offered by paediatric clinical psychologists in hospital include:

- alleviation of distress associated with procedures
- management of pain
- management of anxiety

- problems with treatment adherence

- preparation for hospitalization, surgery and painful procedures

- physical disorders where symptoms may be influenced by psychological factors

- chronic paediatric health problems, chronic conditions

- various psychometric and behavioural assessments

- assistance with psychosomatic disorders.

Children's understanding of illness and pain

Children's knowledge and level of understanding of their bodies, what is happening to them and why this is happening, needs to be taken into account when using psychological methods to manage pain.

A full discussion of children's cognitive development and their perception of illness and pain can be found in Chapter 2. Although there is disagreement about the Piagetian model of child development, most theoretical perspectives generally agree that children develop in stages with concepts becoming more advanced as they grow older. Perception of pain is also affected by life experience and circumstances; every child's perception of pain is unique.

The child's involvement in decision-making and his or her competence to give informed consent are also important.[3,4]

- Internationally the United Nations Rights of the Child Convention has focused on this.

- In the United Kingdom these issues have been highlighted in the Family Law Reform Act and the Children Act (1989).[5,6]

- This has implications for treatment.

Perception of pain is influenced by a person's knowledge, behaviour and feelings. In caring for children this means that:

- the meaning of pain to an individual child might either enhance or decrease their ability to tolerate pain

- however inaccurate the belief-system and understanding the child has, these beliefs are valid for the child
- it is important for health care professionals to establish what the child's beliefs are about pain in order to assist in its management
- in assessing the child's concerns the extent to which they can articulate these, and the clinical interviews with children are important
- interviews with children demand sophistication and require careful setting-up so as to avoid leading questions.[7]

Box 8.1 lists the factors that can affect a child's experience of pain.

Box 8.1   Factors that affect a child's pain experience[8]

- Age
- Understanding
- Learning
- Social reinforcement (e.g. home, school, hospital context)
- Helplessness and issues of control
- Culture
- Gender
- Beliefs, attitudes and expectations
- Pain experiences
- Psychological state (e.g. anxiety, depression)
- Family's response to pain

Coping strategies used by children

There are very few children who use self-initiated coping responses.[2]

- Younger children attempt to gain relief from their pain by passive and concrete methods such as medication and the help of parents and medical or nursing staff.

- Older children use more active approaches such as rubbing the affected spot.

- A low use of coping strategies and a high use of avoidant, maladaptive pain usage has been described.[9]

It has been suggested that:

- some children may construe pain or painful procedures as a punishment. Health care professionals should warn the child that a procedure is likely to be painful, explain why it is being undertaken and that pain is not a punishment

- health care professionals need to explore the ideas that a child has concerning the wider meaning of pain and its implications. Health care professionals should explain in ways the child will understand that pain messages might be helpful in showing us that something is wrong

- children seldom develop their own coping strategies; this has implications for our treatment and training.[2]

Pain is a stressor that affects and disrupts the child's equilibrium. All children have their own ways of trying to restore this when they are affected by a stressor; this is their own coping style. Coping styles are affected by:

- interpersonal resources

- developmental level

- personality

- the child's background

- the child's experiences.

Specific strategies that can be used to defuse the stressor's effects are *coping strategies* or techniques. These may be externally or internally directed.

- Externally they may be direct actions, for example:
    - towards the environment – preparing against harm
    - devising an escape plan
    - showing avoidant behaviour.

- Internally they may be intrapsychic coping processes for example:
    - attention deployment
    - reappraisal
    - wish-fulfilling fantasy.

- Both externally directed and internally directed aspects can be used to deal with pain.
- First one would need to ask the child questions to explore external sources of pain relief (parents, paediatric staff).
- Subsequently one could ask questions about what the children might have tried to do so that 'it wouldn't hurt so much'.

Measurement of pain

Issues which affect pain measurement include:

- context of the pain
- cultural factors
- maturity
- intellectual development
- experience.

Box 8.2 highlights the factors modifying pain perception.

Box 8.2   Factors that modify pain perception[10]

Situational factors	Behavioural factors	Emotional factors
Expectation	Coping style	Fear
Control	Overt distress	Anger
Relevance	Parental response	Frustration
Noxious stimuli	Individual factors	Pain sensation
	Sex	
	Age	
	Culture	
	Cognitive level	
	Previous pains	
	Family learning	

The use of at least one pain assessment measure or tool is suggested since children's self-reports often do not match with observers' assessments. Box 8.3 provides a summary of the distress and pain measures available for use with children. A detailed discussion of pain assessment tools can be found in Chapters 5 and 6. Care needs to be taken when using physiological measures in isolation as, after a period of time, adaptation takes place and physiological changes no longer occur.[11]

Box 8.3 Summary of distress and pain measures[10]

Physiological methods
   Heart rate
   Palmar sweat response
   Blood pressure
   Endorphin levels

Behavioural methods
   Overt distress scales:

   • procedural behavioural rating scale – revised

   • observational scale of behavioural distress

   • Children's Hospital of Eastern Ontario pain scale

Projective methods
   Colours
   Shapes
   Drawings
   Cartoons

Direct report methods
   Interval scales (faces, poker chips, words)
   Interviews (supplied and generate formats)
   Pain questionnaires:

   • children's comprehensive pain questionnaire

   • Varni–Thompson paediatric pain questionnaire

   Visual analogue scale:

   • pain thermometers

   • Oucher scale

The clinical psychologist's assessment

When making decisions about interventions with children with pain one needs to gather as much information as possible upon which to start forming hypotheses. Sources of information are varied – referral letters, conversations with staff and carers, ward reviews and meetings.

The clinical psychologist needs to develop a picture of the child's pain experience and general psychological state based upon thorough assessment and awareness of any problems within the family, such as conflict between divorced parents on the ward.

The child who is referred with a pain problem needs to be seen as a whole person. The following questions can be considered:

- do we focus on the pain symptoms?

- what about an overall assessment?

- do we have an obligation or responsibility to explore problems in the family or parental sub-system?

- have all likely physical 'causes' been investigated thoroughly?

- are these being treated concurrently or have they been excluded?

Basic to all interviews are accurate empathy, non-possessive warmth, genuineness and congruence.[12] Relationships between children and clinical psychologists can be improved through play engagement, the use of projective techniques, open-ended questions and the use of drawings.

Practical applications to assist with paediatric pain

Practical interventions relate to the referral problems that might focus on different types of pain:

- acute pain, which implies pain that is of short duration and that may be associated with a particular condition or treatment procedure

- pain associated with a hurt leg, laceration, or an invasive medical procedure. There may be pain for a protracted period

- chronic pain conditions, over the long term, are an important area for psychological intervention. Such pain may be associated with illnesses such as arthritis and cancer

- psychosomatic pain,* which is usually labelled as such as a result of there not being an obvious organic cause. Although the diagnosis is almost always by exclusion, and there is an emphasis on the 'psychological', this may not be as simple as it appears at first.

Pain is not an 'either/or' concept; the psychological and the physical are inextricably interwoven, and emotion and biology are mutually influencing. Examples where this is often the case include:

- recurrent abdominal pain

- headaches

- earaches of long-standing duration.

Psychological interventions

Psychological applications aim to assist the child and family to deal with the types of problems described above. Issues of self-esteem, depression and coping might be suitably dealt with by psychotherapy, cognitive-behavioural therapy and counselling approaches.

- Where issues concern having procedures which are distressing and sticking to a treatment regime, the child might need a window of space and time to reflect on the situation without pressure.

- It is beneficial to have a person who does not have a medical or nursing role within the multi-disciplinary team to help the child to cope with this.

- The psychologist may be able to examine, together with the child, the child's views about the particular treatment and its effects, as well as the benefits and difficulties associated with treatment; for example, needles, dressings, going to theatre.

- Personal construct psychology can be productively applied to access the child's perspective using a range of techniques.[13,14]

- Issues of consent to treatment are central in this.[15]

- The paediatric psychologist can be a confidant, supporter and advocate for the child.

* *Psychosomatic* does not mean that the pain is not real or 'all in the mind' but can relate to a pain resulting from damage which, having been healed, is intractable. This raises wider issues of perceptions and family dynamics.

Psychological interventions may be from a variety of approaches, yet the central tenet should be that the child has a sense of control from which self-management develops leading to a greater sense of empowerment, confidence and self-efficacy.

As the child feels more competent and able to affect change, the positive cycle develops. Getting this right requires considerable planning and preparation.

'Whatever the behavioural interventions selected, it is vital to convey to the child (and family) that the *child* is acquiring a new skill and heightened control which they can then execute in a situation over which control has to be relinquished. The adult becomes not yet another person doing something *to* children but someone who can help them help themselves to acquire new skills, of which they can be proud.'[2]

A number of procedures and approaches to assist the young person in the self-management process have been described.[2] These include:

- permission to make a noise
- participation
- distraction
- desensitization
- modelling
- cognitive-behavioural interventions
- relaxation
- hypnosis
- guided imagery.

The environment in which treatment takes place provides both challenges and opportunities for professional staff.

- For children and families it may represent a hostile or frightening environment, or it may be judged to be a place where there is treatment expertise and reassurance.
- Staff knowledge, attitudes and practice play an important role in providing an all-round multi-faceted treatment environment.

- Interactions and interrelationships are important and alliances between staff, between staff and patients and within the family have repercussions throughout.

> Children do not necessarily develop ways of dealing with pain by themselves. Few children have natural coping skills. Therefore, these skills need to be taught so that they become integrated as natural mechanisms for coping.

Teaching children these skills is the role of the clinical psychologist. The clinical psychologist can also examine the underlying dynamics and family relationships. Issues in the treatment context as well as pain-focused features must all be incorporated when formulating a treatment plan.

The decision to use psychological or pharmacological approaches, or both, will depend on:

- knowledge of the procedure

- an understanding of the child

- the expectations of pain and anxiety for the child undergoing that procedure.

Types of intervention

Preparation

This is one of the most common types of intervention, and can be undertaken at different levels. Box 8.4 outlines what preparation may involve.

Box 8.4   What preparation involves

- Giving the child information on what is to be done

- Letting the child handle equipment

- The child practising the procedure on a doll

- Introducing the child to the staff

- Discussing fears, feelings and questions that the child may have

---

Preparation is providing information to the child concerning aspects of the impending medical procedure.

- Information concerning the effects on the child's senses in particular should be given, for example touch – if something will be cold.

- The underlying rationale is that unexpected stress is more anxiety-provoking and difficult to deal with than anticipated or predictable stress.

- Information is usually sensory and procedural describing various sensations (touch, sounds, smells, sensations) and outlining steps in the procedure.

It is also important to prepare the child's main carer, particularly as he or she is likely to be present during a medical procedure. The carer may also benefit from learning various anxiety management techniques, and from learning how to coach the child in various simple psychological coping strategies.

Physically focused interventions

Here consideration is given to breathing, relaxation exercises and various forms of distraction. The child is helped to see the relationship between anxiety and physiological signs, and the effect that this has on pain.

- The way in which pain is soothed or relieved when the body is relaxed and floppy is evidence that there is a complex network of interrelationships between *psyche* and *soma*.

- Through the use of a physical strategy, the child is helped to process different modalities selectively. This reframes or distracts from the pain stimulus.

Cognitive-behavioural interventions

These include interventions such as reframing, shaping and rewarding behaviours that one would like to maintain, and desensitization and positive reinforcement regarding anxiety-provoking stimuli.

- Desensitization involves a gradual exposure to things that frighten the child, and positive reinforcement involves giving the child a meaningful reward after the child has exhibited positive coping behaviours.

- Despite their apparent simplicity these procedures require a fair amount of time and planning so that the programme is matched to the individual child.

- The time constraints in the hospital setting usually work against this; these procedures can be effective when linked with specific strategies to help the child cope better.

Children's thoughts, knowledge, expectancies, self-statements, appraisals and the images associated with their behaviour form the focus of this form of intervention. It is considered that beliefs affect stress reactions and that the modification or adaptation of thoughts can help reduce distress. Forms of cognitive-behavioural intervention include:

- thought-stopping, where children can recite a set of clear positive statements when they start thinking about a dreaded procedure

- attention–distraction techniques, where the child can focus on a breathing exercise during the procedure

- reward and incentives, whereby positive reinforcement is used and children are given a trophy or reward after 'doing the best that they could possibly do'

- imagery, where fantasy figures or places are woven into the current medical situation

- behavioural rehearsal, where the child is allowed to play or demonstrate the use of medical/nursing materials

- parents as coaches, affording them a level of control too.

All of these interventions aim to encourage mastery over difficult situations, where children begin to feel that they are successful and thereby increase their self-esteem, control and feeling of self-efficacy.

Applied psychophysiology

In dealing with the child's anxiety about invasive procedures (for example, needles) use can be made of various types of imagery and calming procedures. The use of applied psychophysiology and biofeedback to reduce stress arising from, amongst other things, chronic illness in children has been described.[16,17] Components of biofeedback are:

- the monitoring of physiological processes via electronic equipment

- external feedback of the processes, which allows the child to learn strategies to control these processes.

Success in helping children to relax is associated with their ability automatically to adjust their arousal levels up or down to deal with the stress being encountered. The quieting reflex has been taught extensively to children in schools in the US.[17]

Decreasing the child's hypervigilance associated with negative experiences and helping to relieve heightened arousal is helpful when the child is anxious.

- These techniques may be taught to children as young as three years old to encourage deep breathing and distraction.[18]

- It is possible to give a child a sense of control over events, and help to connote positively some of the situations that are feared.[2]

- Approaches such as hypnotherapy or biofeedback can also be useful for conditioned anxiety states.

With children using computers in educational settings and at home, it is natural to try to match therapeutic material with their aptitude and interests.

- Procedures from psychophysiology and biofeedback are particularly suited to the child's circumstances in the form of computer games.

- In doing this the child's arousal or stress level can be made visible through the application of appropriate equipment.

- Computers and the application of interactive computer software are being used to assist with the stresses associated with procedures, especially haemodialysis.

- This allows children to have a sense of control over their responses, while simultaneously being distracted from the invasive procedures.

- As the skills are internalized, the child gains a sense of self-efficacy and becomes more empowered, thus decreasing the focus or concern about needling or fistula access.

- One such computer programme developed by Ultramind Ltd (London) is called Inner Tuner™, which uses electro-dermal activity or galvanic skin response linked with images on the screen, which the child can modify through learning to control their level of physiological arousal.[19]

- The use of this programme has been evaluated with children on haemodialysis to assist with their adherence around fistula access.[20]

- Indications are that the Inner Tuner™ programme allows for easy engagement of the child and the generalizing of skills learned from interactive software, thereby fostering procedural coping and adherence to treatment.[19]

Hypnosis and guided fantasy/imagery

This is one of the most tested interventions, particularly for use with bone marrow aspirations and lumbar punctures in North America where anaesthetic use is not customary with these procedures. Hypnosis is allied with other cognitive-behavioural strategies and includes deep muscle relaxation and hypnotic suggestions that are built on a base of guided fantasy.

Time optimization for preparation

What is the optimum time for preparation, and how much time should children be given to prepare themselves for an invasive procedure? Too little time and preparation can mean higher levels of distress and anxiety; however, too much time can also result in increased anxiety. Participation can easily slip into prevarication, with an elevation of anxiety and distress. Box 8.5 demonstrates the relationship between anxiety and the time prior to the procedure when the preparation is given.

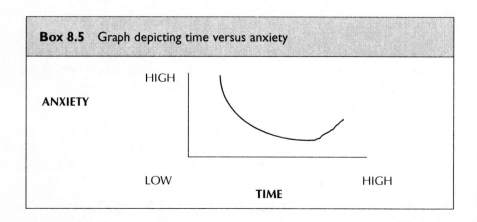

Box 8.5   Graph depicting time versus anxiety

Protocols for assessment and intervention

In working within a paediatric setting it is useful to have standardized protocols and procedures in the management of particular problems. With the management of pain the protocol needs to be adapted and modified for each child. Individual protocols may be developed for a variety of procedures, as well as for children of different ages. An example of a protocol can be seen in Box 8.6.

Box 8.6   An example protocol

Aims/goal: To minimize distress during an invasive medical procedure (IMP).

Process: A step-by-step programme to deal with fear and anxieties and to encourage self-coping behaviours.

Sequence: A series of steps designed for use before, leading up to, during and after the invasive procedure.

(i) Before: Weeks or days before procedure is planned.

(ii) Preceding: Hours or minutes before procedure.

(iii) During: While procedure is undertaken.

(iv) After: Immediate and long-term reinforcement, reward etc.

Before IMP	Preceding IMP	During IMP	After IMP
With the child/ parents/staff			
An ongoing process of:	Preparation	Continuous use of coping strategies	Reward
Education	Listening to the child or young person	Guidelines for staff and/or parents to be more or less active, or not to put pressure on the child	Positive reinforcement
Evaluation			Self-statements
Assessment of experience (past and present)	Practice exercises		Debriefing with staff as well as parents and the young person
Discussion of management	Time limits agreed	Who is present or not present to be agreed	
	Set choices		

Box 8.6   Continued

Before IMP	Preceding IMP	During IMP	After IMP
With the individual child			
Coping technique	Self-in-control via	Measurement using	
Exercises and modelling	– breathing exercises	observational measure of distress, scales etc.	
	– relaxation		
	– imagery		
	– psychophysiology		
	– biofeedback		
	– equipment etc.		
	– plan of action		
Monitoring	Assessment		
Feedback			
e.g. reframing of difficulties, exploring beliefs in self, highlighting successes etc.			

Checklist of issues relating to psychological involvement

A mnemonic may be used to focus on core issues of the clinical psychologist's role in paediatric pain management, which include the following: needs, interventions, time, plan, involvement and communication – 'NITPIC' (Box 8.7).

The role of the clinical psychologist is central to the implementation of psychological methods of pain relief. Psychological methods are particularly useful in chronic pain but their use is not limited to this area.

Box 8.7   Checklist of issues relating to psychological involvement

NEEDS: What does this young person need?
- Being told things
- Being listened to
- Treated with respect
- Reassured
- Offered strategies
- Assessment of their resources

INTERVENTIONS: Which interventions should be used?
- Pharmacological – drugs and dosage ...
- Psychological – approaches, presentation and sequence ...
- Both
- Neither

TIME: What about time constraints?
Decisions about time needed:
- For planning
- For discussions
- For interventions
- For feedback

PLAN: What is the plan of action?
- Availability of resources
- Strategies considered
- Framework established
- Decisions on implementation

INVOLVEMENT: Who is involved?
- Parents
- Medical staff
- Other professionals
- Siblings
- Others

COMMUNICATION: What is this like?
- With the young person, family, siblings
- Within the team/unit/trust
- With colleagues working directly
- Negotiation about roles and functions
- Dealing with anxiety in patient and self

Summary

- There are a number of factors that play a role in diminishing anxiety and distress surrounding painful procedures in paediatrics.

- Psychological methods can be used to help the child cope with painful situations including: relaxation, distraction, breathing, desensitization, positive reinforcement, hypnosis, and cognitive imagery.

- All approaches to relief of pain and distress need to be focused and clear.

- The needs of children and their families need to be taken into consideration as well as the options that are available to them.

- The ultimate skill lies not only in the techniques and their application but in the knowledge, professionalism and ethics of the psychologist making decisions about when and where to apply them.

References

1   Jay SM, Elliot CH, Ozolino M *et al.* (1985) Behavioural management of children's distress during painful medical procedures. *Behav Res Ther.* **23** (1): 513–20.
2   Lansdown R and Sokel B (1993) Commissioned review: Approaches to pain management in children. *ACCP Rev.* **15** (3): 105–11.
3   Koocher GP and DeMaso DR (1990) Children's competence to consent to medical procedures. *Paediatrician.* **17**: 68–73.
4   Reissland N (1983) Cognitive maturity and the experience of fear and pain in hospital. *Soc Sci Med.* **17**: 1389–95.
5   HMSO (1969) *The Family Law Reform Act.* HMSO, London.
6   HMSO (1989) *The Children Act.* HMSO, London.
7   Bush JP (1987) Pain in children: a review of the literature from a developmental perspective. *Psychol Health.* **1**: 215–36.
8   McGrath PJ (1989) Evaluating a child's pain. *J Pain Symptom Manage.* **4** (4): 55–63.
9   Ross DM and Ross SA (1984) Childhood pain: the school aged child's viewpoint. *Pain.* **20**: 179–91.
10 McGrath PJ (1990) *Pain in Children: Nature, Assessment and Treatment.* Guildford Publications, New York.
11 Gildea JH, Quirk JH and Quirk TH (1977) Assessing the pain experience in children. *Nurs Clin North Am.* **1**: 631–7.
12 Rogers C (1951) *Client-Centred Therapy: Its Current Practice, Implications and Theory.* Houghton Mifflin, Boston.
13 Butler RJ (1985) Towards an understanding of childhood difficulties. In: *Reperatory Grids and Personal Constructs* (ed. N Beail). Croom Holm, London.
14 Ravenette AT (1980) *The Exploration of Consciousness: Personal Construct Psychology, Psychotherapy and Personality.* Wiley, New York.
15 Alderson P (1990) Choosing for children: Parents consent to surgery. In: *Working With Families of Children With Special Needs* (ed N Dale). Routledge, London.

16 Gagnon DJ, Hudnall L and Andrasik F (1992) Biofeedback and related procedures in coping with stress. In: *Stress and Coping in Child Health* (eds AM La Greca, LJ Siegal, JL Wallander *et al*.). Guildford Press, New York.

17 Stroebel E and Stroebel CF (1984) The quieting reflex: a psychophysiological approach for helping children deal with healthy and unhealthy stress. In: *Stress and Coping in Child Health* (eds AM La Greca, LJ Siegal, JL Wallander *et al*.). Guildford Press, New York.

18 Kuttner L (1989) Management of children's acute pain and anxiety during invasive medical procedure. *Paediatrician.* **16**: 39–44.

19 Ultramind Ltd, Inner Tuner ™ *Integrated psychological and applied psychophysiological systems approach to well being through health psychology.* Multimedia Interactive Software, London.

20 Morris T and Lawson A (1997) *Preparing children for renal dialysis.* Presentation at the Third Research Fair in Child and Adolescent Mental Health, Parkview Clinic, University of Birmingham, March 1997.

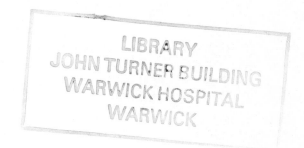

9 The pharmacological management of acute pain

Introduction

The report *Pain After Surgery* criticized the management of post-operative pain relief.[1] In 1996, Cummings *et al.* found that children are still experiencing unacceptable levels of pain during hospitalization.[2] This is due to a number of factors, one of which is the lack of knowledge among medical and nursing staff regarding the use of analgesics. This chapter will discuss the pharmacological methods available for the management of acute pain in children. The need for a clinical protocol will be discussed, and the benefits of an acute pain team presented.

Standardization of analgesia

In order to simplify the prescription of analgesia, only four drugs are required:

- paracetamol
- diclofenac
- codeine phosphate
- morphine.

With these four drugs, a simple but flexible analgesic ladder can be produced (Figure 9.1). Doses for these four drugs are shown in Box 9.1.

The combination of an analgesic ladder and the guide to drug doses will allow medical and nursing staff to make informed and effective decisions about the prescription of analgesia.

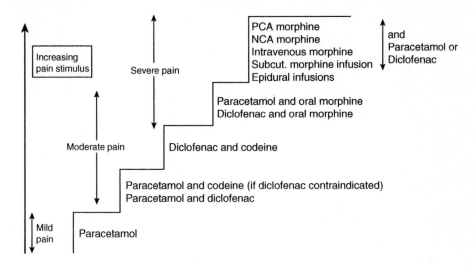

Figure 9.1:   A simple analgesic ladder.

General principles

Assessment of the child

Before implementing a pain management strategy, a history of the child's previous experiences of pain needs to be obtained. This pain history will include:

- the responses of the child to pain
- a history of previous pain experiences
- the words used by the child to describe pain
- the reactions of the child to pain
- methods used to comfort the child when in pain.

It is also important to consider the type, site and duration of any pain, as well as the developmental stage of the child. At this time the nurse or doctor should determine any anxieties the child or family may have.

Box 9.1 Drug doses

Drug	Dose by mouth	Dose rectally	Dose intra-muscularly or intravenous bolus	Dose by infusion
Paracetamol	15–20 mg/kg 4-hourly	35 mg/kg 4-hourly	Not available yet	Not available
Diclofenac	1 mg/kg 8-hourly	1 mg/kg 8-hourly	Not available	Not available
Codeine phosphate	1 mg/kg 4-hourly	1 mg/kg 4-hourly	1 mg/kg 4-hourly	Contraindicated
Morphine sulphate:				
• children > 6 months of age	0.1–0.2 mg/kg 4-hourly	0.1–0.2 mg/kg 4-hourly	0.1–0.2 mg/kg 4-hourly	5–30 μg/kg/hr (1 mg/kg of morphine sulphate in 50 ml of solution produces a concentration of 20 μg/kg thus 1 ml/hr = 20 μg/kg/hr)
• children < 6 months of age	0.1 mg/kg 8-hourly	0.1 mg/kg 8-hourly	0.1 mg/kg 8-hourly	5–10 μg/kg/hr
• children on ventilatory support	Not applicable	Not applicable	0.1 mg/kg 4-hourly	5–60 μg/kg/hr

Once a pain history has been taken, the multi-disciplinary team, in conjunction with the child and family, should devise a pain management strategy. This will incorporate:

- the various analgesics required
- the method of delivery of analgesics, for example intravenous, epidural, patient controlled analgesia (PCA)
- the benefits of each regimen
- the possible side effects, and methods of relieving these side effects
- monitoring requirements
- methods for the family to obtain advice from medical and nursing staff.

Information given to the child, and parents, at this time can be reinforced by the use of information leaflets.

Pain assessment

This has been covered in Chapter 5. It is important that children have their pain assessed and reassessed at regular intervals and that the effectiveness of pain-relieving strategies is evaluated.

Non-drug methods of analgesia

Non-drug methods of analgesia must be used in conjunction with any analgesic agents required. (*See* Chapter 7 for further discussion on non-drug methods of pain relief.)

Analgesic drugs

These may be divided into three groups:

- non-opioid drugs:
  - paracetamol
  - non-steroidal anti-inflammatory drugs (NSAIDs)
- opioids, and opioid delivery systems
- local anaesthetic agents and techniques.

Non-opioid analgesics

Paracetamol. The commonest agent prescribed for analgesia in children, this is effective as a sole agent only for mild pain and is still used inappropriately when pain increases.

- It is not yet clear how paracetamol produces analgesia but it is thought that by inhibition of prostaglandin synthesis in the brain it impairs the perception of pain.

- Because of this site of action paracetamol will produce a much greater effect when used in conjunction with NSAIDs than when used alone.

- Paracetamol has little anti-inflammatory activity, despite being effective in juvenile rheumatoid arthritis, and has little anti-platelet activity.

- Oral paracetamol is dependent on normal gastrointestinal function for its absorption and so is ineffective after major surgery; in this situation, rectal paracetamol is available (Box 9.1).

- Suppositories should only be administered after obtaining consent from the child and family.

Non-steroidal anti-inflammatory drugs (NSAIDs). Over recent years there has been a rapid increase in the use of NSAIDs for analgesia.

- NSAIDs act by the inhibition of prostaglandin synthesis.

- Prostaglandins have a number of actions in the body.

- In relation to pain management they are important in the production of the pain impulse, by sensitizing the nerve endings to the effect of brady-kinin, a substance released by tissues when pain stimuli are produced.

- Prostaglandins are present in both peripheral and central nerves, however the predominant site of action is peripheral, thus, prostaglandins complement the effects of paracetamol and opioids, which act on the central nervous system.

- NSAIDs have an onset of action of more than 20 minutes, and thus to be effective need to be administered before procedures begin.

The side effects of NSAIDs are also due to prostaglandin inhibition:

- decrease in platelet activity
- increase in the incidence of gastrointestinal bleeding
- decrease in renal blood flow, and impaired renal function.

These side effects are less frequent in children.[4] NSAIDs are, however, contraindicated in the following patients:

- patients with renal impairment
- hypovolaemic patients
- patients with a tendency to bleed:
  - haemophilia
  - bone marrow depression
  - low platelet count (<100 000)
- patients with liver disease
- children under six months of age
- gastrointestinal ulceration.

The allergic hypersensitivity syndrome that is seen with aspirin is not seen with NSAIDs, thus, these drugs are not contraindicated in patients with asthma. However, because of prostaglandin inhibition, there may be a worsening of asthma symptoms and NSAIDs should only be administered to asthmatic children under medical supervision, and parents should be warned about the possible increase in frequency of symptoms of asthma.

Diclofenac (oral and rectal administration) and *ketorolac* (0.5 mg/kg intravenous administration) are useful in mild to moderate pain.

- Ideally these are used in conjunction with other analgesics, such as paracetamol or opioids.
- Diclofenac is now available as a dispersible solution, allowing a 1 mg/kg dose prescription for all children.
- Useful as a supplement to other forms of analgesia such as PCA or epidural infusions.

Opioid analgesics

Codeine phosphate

- Codeine has one sixth the activity of morphine and, as a consequence, a lower incidence of respiratory depression.
- It is best used in conjunction with NSAIDs or paracetamol for moderate pain.
- If patients are unable to tolerate morphine for severe pain, then the combination of regular codeine and NSAIDs may be a suitable alternative.

- Codeine should *never* be given intravenously as it may produce apnoea and severe hypotension.[5]

- In pre-term infants it may still produce respiratory depression and apnoeic episodes and its use then should be carefully monitored with oxygen saturation monitors.

A side effect of codeine phosphate is constipation; a stool softener, such as lactulose, should be prescribed and when possible a high fibre diet encouraged.

Morphine sulphate. Despite advances in pain assessment and delivery systems, morphine remains the drug of choice for severe pain. With increasing frequency of usage, and the production of protocols, medical and nursing staff have become more confident in the use of morphine for both children and neonates. Box 9.2 lists the advantages and disadvantages of the different routes of administration of morphine and identifies when it is appropriate to use each route.

Patient controlled analgesia (PCA)

Analgesic requirements are not constant and this has led to the introduction and increasing acceptance of PCA.[6] It is a highly effective method of administering analgesia intravenously.

- The use of bolus doses of analgesic administered by the patient allows children more control over their pain medication, allowing the delivery of analgesia to coincide with any pain.

- PCA morphine in children produces the same analgesic effect as intramuscular injections but with less sedation.[7]

- Adult PCA regimens do not translate in paediatric practice; PCA with a low background infusion (4 μg/kg/h) has better pain scores and sleep patterns, less nausea and vomiting and less respiratory depression than PCA with either no background infusion or a high background infusion (10 μg/kg/h).[8]

- The treatment regimen advocated by Lloyd-Thomas and Howard can be seen in Box 9.3.[9]

- The use of PCA requires thorough education of the child and family in order to be effective.

- This preferably occurs before any pain stimulus.

- The child must be educated in the use of the 'button' controlling the device before pain occurs or before any painful procedure.

Box 9.2   Morphine administration

Route	Advantages	Disadvantages	Uses
Oral	• easy administration • well tolerated • simple formulation	• not effective if patient has nausea or vomiting • onset of 20 minutes, therefore, timing of administration is important • produces fluctuations in analgesic level	• acute, severe pain • bone fractures and manipulation of fractures • change of dressings
Rectal	• effective if patient is vomiting • easy administration	• not liked by children • fluctuations in analgesic level	• after major surgery
Intra-muscular	• none, unless patient is anaesthetized when it may produce an awake comfortable child after surgery	• children hate injections and thus intra-muscular morphine should not be used unless the child is anaesthetized	• ENT surgery • neurosurgery
Subcutaneous	• continuous administration • does not need intravenous access	• amount of drug delivered is dependent on tissue perfusion thus the possibility of overdosage after a period of poor tissue perfusion	• cancer pain • post-operatively in children with poor veins
Intravenous	• continuous administration • less variable analgesic level • allows drug boluses to be added • level of analgesic more easily controlled	• requires intravenous access • requires special monitoring (respiratory rate, pulse oximetry) • drug level does not change quickly enough to new effective level (see PCA)	• any inpatient with severe pain

Box 9.3 Infusion guidelines for PCA and NCA
(adapted from Lloyd-Thomas and Howard with permission)[9]

Techniques	Standard infusions
PCA	Morphine sulphate 1 mg/kg in 50 ml 5% glucose = 20 µg/kg/ml Maximum 4-hourly dose = 400 µg/kg
NCA	Morphine sulphate 1 mg/kg in 50 ml 5% glucose = 20 µg/kg/ml Maximum 4-hourly dose = 400 µg/kg
Subcutaneous PCA/NCA	Morphine sulphate 1 mg/kg in 20 ml normal saline = 50 µg/kg/ml Maximum 4-hourly dose = 400 µg/kg

Initial programming	Loading dose		Background infusion		Bolus dose		Lockout
	µg/kg	ml	µg/kg/hr	ml/hr	µg/kg	ml	min
PCA	50–100	2.5–5	2–8	0.1–0.4	10–20	0.5–1	5–15
NCA	50–100	2.5–5	10–20	0.5–1	10–20	0.5–1	30–60

- It is important to continue to reassure the child and reinforce information regularly, especially in the period after initiating the device, when the child's and parents' fear and anxiety about analgesic failure are greatest.

- Children above seven years of age are able to understand the use of PCA; children under five cannot.

- Children aged five to seven years represent a group of patients in whom PCA may be used, but they require more reassur-ance and education, and in this group a combination of PCA and NCA is better.[9]

- This is especially useful after surgery, when children initially receive NCA as they are still sedated from the anaesthetic and unable to use PCA, but after a day they are more aware, and the infusion is changed to PCA.

- If the child is in pain at the start of PCA a loading dose must be administered to ensure an adequate drug level in the body.

Nurse controlled analgesia (NCA)

In children under five years of age the use of NCA has become popular.[9] This is essentially a morphine infusion with the ability to administer controlled boluses of the drug at times of increased pain.

- To prevent an overdose of morphine a longer lockout time is employed.

- Parents are consulted about the need for extra analgesia but it is the responsibility of the nurse to administer the drug.

- If the child is in pain at the start of NCA a loading dose must be administered to ensure an adequate drug level in the body.

PCA and NCA may be administered by indwelling subcutaneous catheters, when the concentration should be increased to 50 micrograms/ml. The feeling of the delivery of drug by this method may produce an increase in placebo effect, and therefore better pain scores.[9]

Side effects of morphine

When intravenous preparations of morphine are used, and especially PCA or NCA, the amount of drug delivered to the child is higher than with regular intra-muscular injections. This produces better pain scores but also an increase in side effects.

NAUSEA AND VOMITING

Some children dislike the presence of nausea and vomiting so much that they prefer mild discomfort and do not press a PCA button. Ondansetron seems to be the most effective anti-emetic, at present, and can be added to the morphine infusion.

RESPIRATORY DEPRESSION

This is always a concern with morphine infusions and strict monitoring and protocols are required to prevent it. The presence of increasing sedation is an indicator of impending respiratory depression. The use of pre-printed prescription charts with dosages of drugs such as naloxone has increased confidence among medical and nursing staff.

CONSTIPATION

This should be expected with morphine infusions. A stool softener should be prescribed and a high fibre diet should be encouraged.

ITCHING OR URINARY RETENTION

Itching and urinary retention are more common with epidural morphine. They may cause distress to the child, and the use of low dose naloxone (up to 2 μg/kg) or chlorpheniramine (0.1 mg/kg) may be required. If naloxone is not effective, then the epidural infusion may need to be stopped and an alternative method of analgesia instituted.

Morphine in neonates

Neonates are more sensitive than children to the effects of morphine because they have:

- a higher level of natural endogenous opioids, which decreases morphine requirements

- an incomplete blood-brain barrier, so more administered drug reaches the brain[10]

- a greater variation in opiate receptor types, with an increase in respiratory depression receptors[11]

- less ability to bind morphine to plasma proteins, increasing the amount of free drug in the body[12]

- less ability to metabolize and excrete morphine, so the drug stays in the body longer.[13]

The use of morphine in neonates is thus more variable in its effects than in children, the dose needs to be reduced to 5–10 μg/kg/h, and the neonate needs to be observed closely with pulse oximetry for any signs of respiratory depression.

Local anaesthetic agents and techniques

Local anaesthetics are ideal agents to produce analgesia because they work locally to nerves, are generally safe, and may produce long-lasting complete analgesia of the affected parts of the body. This facilitates the discharge of a pain-free and alert child after day surgery.

- Local anaesthetics decrease the need for other analgesics with a resultant decrease in side effects.

- Decreasing the requirement for opioids may improve respiratory function, which may be critical in some patients.

- Local anaesthetics may be used on a single occasion (for example when blocking the nerves of a finger) or, with the improvement in catheter design, may be administered by infusion to maintain analgesia for a number of days (for example in epidural infusions).

Local anaesthetics may be divided structurally into two groups, amides and esters (Box 9.4).

Amide local anaesthetics:

- are more stable in solution

- produce less anaphylaxis

- are metabolized in the liver.

Ester local anaesthetics are metabolized in the liver and plasma by cholinesterase enzymes.

- In children, a greater percentage of body weight is produced by water and as local anaesthetics stay in the body water compartment, they may be used in bigger initial doses than in adults.

- Children clear local anaesthetic drugs from the body faster than adults, and so tolerate higher infusion rates.

- Neonates clear local anaesthetics less well, and so infusion rates need to be reduced in order to prevent accumulation and toxicity.[14]

Local anaesthetic agents work by inhibiting the entry of sodium ions into nerves, and thus need to be deposited at the site of the nerves. There are a number of methods available to do this, either in the region of peripheral nerves (Box 9.5) or around nerves as they leave the spine.

CAUDAL EPIDURAL ANALGESIA

In children caudal epidural techniques are simple to perform (Figure 9.2) and as they produce effective, long-lasting analgesia they are used frequently.

Box 9.4 Peripheral nerve blocks

Drugs	Advantages	Disadvantages	Uses
Amides			
Lignocaine	• faster onset • less cardiotoxic in overdose	• short duration • decreases movement of area	• urethral catheterization • finger blocks • insertion of indwelling lines
Prilocaine	• fast onset • least cardiotoxic in overdose	metabolized by the liver to a substance which may be toxic in young children	Biers blocks in older children
Bupivacaine	• long duration • allows mobilization	• most cardiotoxic in overdose • needs to be used by infusion in conjunction with opiate	operative and post-operative analgesia
Ropivacaine	• long duration • allows more mobilization • may be used as sole agent • safer than bupivacaine	• new agent	may supersede bupivacaine as agent for infusions
Esters			
Amethocaine	• absorbed easily through the skin • vasodilates surface veins	• irritant if left on the skin too long	topical analgesia (Ametop)
Cocaine	• well absorbed	• toxicity	eye anaesthesia

Box 9.5   Topical blocks

Nerve block	Examples	Advantages	Disadvantages	Uses
Skin (topical)	EMLA cream	• absorbed by the skin	• requires 1 hour to be effective	• cannulation of veins • insertion of drains • minor surgery to the skin
	Ametop cream	• faster (30 minutes) onset than EMLA • longer duration of action (even if removed) • vasodilates veins making cannulation easier	• more irritant to the skin • more expensive	• cannulation of veins • insertion of drains • minor surgery to the skin
	Lignocaine cream Lignocaine spray	• fastest onset • may be applied to mucous membranes	• short duration • rapid absorption and thus higher plasma levels	• urethral catheter insertion • anaesthesia of the larynx
Nerve blocks	Arm, leg, fingers, toes	• simple, produce complete anaesthesia • reduce the need for opioids	• none	• surgery on the described regions
	Inguinal, intercostal and penile blocks	• produce long-lasting analgesia • reduce the need for opioids	• require specialist for the local anaesthetic to be sited correctly	• herniotomies • circumcision • orchidopexy • appendicectomy

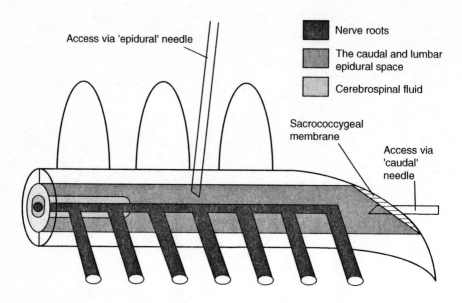

Access via 'epidural' needle

Nerve roots

The caudal and lumbar epidural space

Cerebrospinal fluid

Sacrococcygeal membrane

Access via 'caudal' needle

Figure 9.2: A schematic diagram to demonstrate the methods of access and anatomy of the epidural space.

- Advances in catheter design allow the placement of catheters into the epidural space via the caudal route, generating analgesia for a number of days.

- This is particularly suitable for neonates.

- Bupivacaine is, at present, the drug of choice for caudal analgesia, and the quality and duration of action may be improved by the addition of either morphine, clonidine or ketamine.[15,17]

- The combination of bupivacaine and morphine may produce analgesia for up to 24 hours, but the child needs to be observed closely because of the possibility of respiratory depression.

- Caudal analgesia is less attractive in older children because of the side effect of leg weakness which results in slow mobilization.

- Ropivacaine is a newer drug that is currently being evaluated. This drug produces less leg weakness, and thus earlier mobilization, and may become the drug of choice.

INTERVERTEBRAL EPIDURAL ANALGESIA

Excellent long-term analgesia may be produced by the use of epidural local anaesthetic infusions. The required site of the epidural catheter is determined by the drug being used:

- if *ropivacaine* alone or *fentanyl* is used the catheter needs to be sited at the level of the vertebra closest to the nerves which transmit the pain stimulus

- if *morphine* or *diamorphine* are used with either bupivacaine[18] or ropivacaine, the catheter can be sited away from the dermatomal level, thus reducing the possibility of damage to the spinal cord.

The technique has been simplified by the production of short 18-gauge epidural needles (Portex UK). The dose of local anaesthetic is reduced by the addition of morphine to the infusion. This increases the quality of the analgesia, but also increases the incidence of side effects.

Side effects of epidural infusions are:

- nausea and vomiting, although less than intravenous morphine

- itching

- urinary retention; epidural infusions should only be employed if the child has a urethral catheter as part of the procedure, or if the child's bladder may be expressed by the Crede manoeuvre

- respiratory depression; the incidence is less than with intravenous morphine (as long as the dose of morphine is kept below 5 μg/kg/h or the dose of fentanyl below 0.4 μg/kg/h).[19]

These side effects may be reduced or disappear with the use of ropivacaine, which allows a higher concentration of local anaesthetic to be used, and thus obviates the need for an additional opioid. When using ropivacaine, it is necessary to place the catheter close to the dermatomal level of the pain, and also to administer regular NSAIDs.

Epidural infusions need to be monitored closely; initially there is a failure rate of up to 5%, when the epidural infusion fails to produce adequate analgesia and needs to be stopped. An alternative method of producing analgesia such as PCA should be used. When using an epidural infusion the patient must be closely monitored for pain and sedation scores and the incidence of side effects.

Specific pain management problems

Procedural pain and trauma pain

Intense short-duration pain is very difficult to manage. It requires the use of strong analgesics which are of short- or medium-term duration. The use of strong analgesics results in a number of unwelcome side effects. Timing of the administration of these agents is also important.

- As an adjunct to analgesics, non-drug methods must be employed as fully as possible, with distraction, reassurance and control of analgesia as important facets.

- The use of play therapists at this time is invaluable.

- Topical analgesia is the method of choice because of effectiveness and safety.

- Local anaesthesia may also be used after topical anaesthesia – for example, femoral nerve blockade for femoral fractures.

- Systemic agents (Box 9.6) will, however, be needed in a number of situations.

- Sedative agents such as benzodiazepines will not produce analgesia and cannot be used as sole agents because of the anxiety associated with procedural pain, but are useful when used in conjunction with analgesics. This does, however, increase the incidence of respiratory complications.

- Strict protocols should be available for agents' doses and monitoring.

Day case analgesia

The increase in children treated on a day-case basis has made medical and nursing staff reassess the analgesia given to these patients. As the patient leaves the hospital so soon after surgery, the analgesic plan must be formulated carefully.

- Studies have shown that the first post-operative night is associated with severe pain, especially among patients who have undergone orchidopexy or circumcision.[20,21]

- Local anaesthesia will last for up to eight hours.

- Pain may return after discharge home where often the only analgesic available is paracetamol.

Box 9.6 Analgesics for procedural and trauma pain

Analgesic	Advantages	Disadvantages	Uses
Entonox	• rapid onset • rapid offset • potent • little effect on intracranial pressure	• difficult to synchronize with pain • high incidence of nausea	older children
Oral morphine	• easy administration • easier timing • mildly sedating	• slow onset • nausea and vomiting • less of a peak in analgesia • long duration	medium intensity pain
Intravenous morphine	• simple synchronization with pain	• requires intravenous access • requires respiratory monitors • long duration	high intensity pain
Intravenous fentanyl	• rapid onset • short duration • simple timing	• requires intravenous access • requires respiratory monitoring • very potent	high intensity pain
Ketamine	• a potent analgesic as well as an anaesthetic • less respiratory depression than opioids • minimal cardiovascular depression	• is an anaesthetic and thus requires careful monitoring and staff skilled in airway management • may produce hallucinations and emergence psychosis • increases salivation • increases intracranial pressure	high intensity pain

- The use of diclofenac (1 mg/kg) 8-hourly for the three days after discharge is recommended and should be accompanied by written information.

- All patients who have no contraindication to NSAIDs should be given a three day supply with instructions on frequency of dosage and the use of additional paracetamol, if required.

- The family needs to be able to contact the ward or community paediatric nurses if further information or help is required.

The pain team

The management of pain requires a multi-disciplinary team, which should comprise medical staff, nursing staff, psychologists, play therapists, pharmacists and physiotherapists.

- Central to the group are anaesthetists and nurse specialists who provide a focus for education, problem solving, audit, and research.[22]

- The principal member of the pain team is the nurse looking after the patient; this is the person who delivers the care, and who monitors and adjusts the interventions required to manage pain.

- The management of pain must empower the nurse to this central role.[23]

Pain protocols

A pain protocol allows the simplification and standardization of analgesic policy within a hospital. It should provide all hospital staff with information and guidance on the use of analgesics and methods of administration. It is, therefore, a key element in the provision of effective analgesia to children. The protocol should include:

- analgesic regimens

- monitoring guidelines

- nursing care plans

- nursing standard

- audit methods

- guidelines about specific types of pain:
  - post-operative pain
  - procedural pain

  - acute relapsing pain, e.g. sickle-cell disease
  - cancer pain
  - patients with renal or hepatic impairment
- access to further information:
  - medical staff
  - references
  - further reading.

The protocol should be readily available throughout the hospital.

Having a pain protocol will help to ensure that children no longer endure unnecessary pain.

Summary

- Pain in children has historically always been badly managed.

- This is often due to a lack of knowledge of analgesic agents, fear of over-dosage of drugs or the possibility of producing dependence on opiates.

- It is possible to standardize the prescription of analgesics using four drugs: paracetamol, diclofenac, codeine phosphate and morphine.

- There are a number of different drug delivery devices; each child should have his or her pain assessed and an individual analgesic plan drawn up.

- The combination of an analgesic ladder and a guide to drug dosages will allow informed and effective choices to be made about the prescription of analgesic drugs.

References

1   The Royal College of Surgeons of England and the College of Anaesthetists. Commission on the Provision of Surgical Services (1990) *Report of a working party on pain after surgery.* HMSO, London.
2   Cummings EA, Reid GJ, Finlay A *et al.* (1996) A survey of parent's expectations and perceptions of their children's experiences. *Pain.* **68**: 25–31.
3   Rusy LM, Houck CS, Sullivan LJ *et al.* (1995) A double blind evaluation of ketorolac tromethamine versus acetaminophen in pediatric tonsillectomy: analgesia and bleeding. *Anesth Analg.* **80**: 226.
4   Maunuksela EL, Olkkola KT and Korpela R (1988) Does prophylactic intravenous infusion of indomethacin improve the management of postoperative pain in children? *Can J Anesth.* **35**: 123–7.
5   Yaster M and Deshpande JK (1988) Management of pediatric pain with opioid analgesics. *Pediatrics.* **113**: 421–9.

6   Bray RJ, Woodhams AM, Vallis CJ et al. (1996) A double blind comparison of morphine infusion and patient controlled analgesia in children. Paediatr Anaesth. 6: 121–7.

7   Berde CB, Lehn BN, Yee YD et al. (1993) Patient controlled analgesia in children and adolescents: a randomised prospective comparison with intramuscular morphine for postoperative analgesia. Pediatrics. 118: 460–6.

8   Doyle E, Harper I and Morton NS (1993) Patient Controlled Analgesia with low dose background infusions after lower abdominal surgery in children. Br J Anaesth. 71: 818–22.

9   Lloyd-Thomas AR and Howard RF (1994) A pain service for children. Paediatr Anaesth. 4: 3–15.

10   Kupferburg HJ and Way EL (1963) Pharmacological basis for the increased sensitivity of the rat brain to morphine. J Pharmacol Exp Ther. 141: 105–12.

11   Leslie RM, Tso S and Holbutt TE (1982) Differential appearance of opiate receptor subtypes in the neonatal rat brain. Life Sci. 31: 1393–6.

12   Morselli PI, Franco-Morselli R and Borsi L (1980) Clinical pharmacokinetics in newborns and infants. Age related differences and therapeutic implications. Clin Pharm. 5: 485–527.

13   Lynn AM and Slattery JT (1987) Morphine pharmacokinetics in early pregnancy. Anesthesiology. 66: 136–9.

14   Berde C (1992) Convulsions associated with pediatric regional anaesthesia. Anesth Analg. 75: 164–6.

15   Wolf AR, Hughes D, Wade A et al. (1990) Postoperative analgesia after paediatric orchidopexy: evaluation of a bupivacaine-morphine mixture. Br J Anaesth. 64: 430–5.

16   Lee JI and Rubin AP (1994) Comparison of a bupivacaine-clonidine mixture with plain bupivacaine for caudal analgesia in children. Br J Anaesth. 72: 258–62.

17   Cook B, Grubb DJ, Aldridge LA et al. (1995) Comparison of the effects of adrenaline, clonidine and ketamine on the duration of analgesia produced by bupivacaine in children. Br J Anaesth. 75: 698–701.

18   Krane EJ, Jacobsen LE, Lynn AM et al. (1987) Caudal morphine for postoperative analgesia in children: a comparison with caudal bupivacaine and intravenous morphine. Anesth Analg. 66: 647–53.

19   Berde C (1994) Epidural analgesia in children. Can J Anesth. 41: 555–60.

20   Tan SGM, May HA and Cunliffe M (1994) An audit of pain and vomiting in paediatric day case surgery. Paediatr Anaesth. 4: 105–9.

21   Knight JC (1994) Postoperative pain in children after day case surgery. Paediatr Anaesth. 4: 45–51.

22   Goddard JM and Pickup SE (1996) Postoperative pain in children. Anaesthesia. 51: 588–90.

23   Lloyd-Thomas AR, Howard R and Llewellyn N (1995) The management of acute and postoperative pain in infancy and childhood. In: Baillière's Clinical Paediatrics. Stress and Pain in Infancy and Childhood (guest eds A Aynsley-Green, M Ward-Platt and AR Lloyd-Thomas). WB Saunders, London. 3 (3), 579–99.

10 The management of chronic pain

'Pain is a more terrible Lord of mankind than even death itself' Albert Schweitzer.[1]

Chronic pain in children is a very different subject from its adult counterpart; in particular degenerative conditions do not feature and the psychological 'baggage' of adulthood has not been accumulated. The management of children with chronic pain can be more difficult for several other reasons:

- age – the perception and expression of pain changes with age and experience

- cause – pain associated with childhood cancer may be associated with much anxiety for patient and family

- severity – long-term unremitting pain, as may occur with arthritis, may require as much psychological input in treatment as pharmacological input

- the family – a child with a chronic illness of any sort will cause added strains within the family context and, therefore, pain management will need to include the family in its entirety. Much of a health care professional's time may be spent explaining the role of controlling a child's pain within the context of treating the illness as a whole.

This chapter will present an overview of current practice by discussing methods of treatment in general, and then this will be applied by looking at several conditions that can result in chronic pain in children.

The International Association for the Study of Pain (IASP) defines pain as: 'An unpleasant, sensory and emotional experience associated with actual or potential tissue damage or described in terms of such damage'.

There are several points to note about this definition:

- the experience of pain is subjective and therefore individual
- the psychological impact cannot be separated from the sensation
- the response to pain depends on previous experience.

This last point is of particular relevance when dealing with a paediatric population whose experience of their environment and bodies varies widely with age and is changing rapidly.

The term 'chronic' pain equates in the minds of many with pain that is not acute or severe. This is not always the case. For instance, in sickle cell crises the pain can be both acute and severe. In addition, pain can persist beyond any evidence of ongoing tissue damage, as in sympathetically mediated pain syndromes; this pain is caused by damage to the sympathetic nervous system, which results in the normal flow of efferent sympathetic activity leading to the abnormal sensation of pain long after the initial painful event has passed. An example of this would be a sympathetic dystrophy.

Chronic pain is, therefore, defined as: 'Pain which persists beyond the usual course of an acute disease or which is associated with an underlying chronic condition'.[2]

When considering how to treat pain it is important to have tried to ascertain the cause of the pain. A good history is vitally important, supported by a physical examination and appropriate investigations.

- The nature of the pain should be determined, using language that may be understood by the child. In this context it should be remembered that children in pain may show signs of regression. (*See* Chapter 2 for a discussion of children's cognitive level and their perception of pain.)

- Note should be made of recent analgesic interventions and how well they are controlling pain as this may give clues to disease progression or the development of tolerance to drugs that have been used over a long period.

- The psychological impact of the diagnosis on the patient and the family should be assessed as this may alter the severity of the painful experience.

- Finally some assessment of potential routes for the administration of analgesics should be considered.

When considering a treatment strategy:

- one should aim to manage the pain adequately whilst avoiding, as far as possible, significant side effects. This balance is different for each child and any regimen must be tailored to fit the individual's needs

- associated problems need to be anticipated and addressed at an early stage; for example, laxatives should be given to a child on strong opioids

- discussion with the family and child should take place to dispel any fears and misconceptions that either may have. This is particularly true if the child requires strong opioids as there is a general, if largely overplayed, fear of dependence and addiction.

Pain control can be provided by pharmacological and non-drug methods.

Pharmacological treatment

Good pain management depends on:

- the use of appropriate drugs
- at appropriate dosage
- via an appropriate route
- at appropriate frequencies.

In adult pain management the concept of an analgesic ladder is adopted; this approach is equally valid with children, although the route may be slightly different.[3]

The analgesic drugs available fall into three categories and are listed in Box 10.1.

> Having decided on an appropriate drug(s), thought must be given to the most appropriate *route* of delivery.

The routes available are:

- enteral (PO or PR) – the most non-invasive route
- transdermal – fentanyl patches are available and have been used for treating cancer pain in adults.[4] Although they bridge the gap between

Box 10.1 Classification of analgesic drugs

Drug class	Drug	Dose and route	Problems
Non-opioids	Paracetamol	15 mg/kg PO 6-hourly 20 mg/kg PR 8-hourly	Rare mainly of overdose
	NSAIDs		Gastric irritation May worsen asthma Nephrotoxicity
Weak opioids	Codeine	1 mg/kg PO, PR, SC, IM 6-hourly	Constipation
	Buprenorphine	3–9 μg/kg SC, IM, IV	Partial agonist therefore ceiling effect may be a problem
Strong opioids	Morphine	No maximum limit to dose PO, SC, IM, IV, (spinal, epidural)	Sedation, respiratory depression, nausea, constipation etc.
	Methadone	100–200 μg/kg PO, SC, IM	As for morphine Long half-life may be advantageous especially for overnight dosing

enteral and parenteral (IM and IV) administration of strong opiates they
have a number of disadvantages:
- fixed strength (25, 50, 75, 100 μg/hr)
- slow onset times due to the drug having to diffuse into and through
  the dermis
- slow offset times because the dermis acts as a reservoir for the drug;
  it may take up to 17 hours for the plasma concentration to fall by
  half.

These properties preclude the use of fentanyl patches in paediatrics:

- intra-muscular (IM) route – offers unpredictable levels of analgesia and
  holds such dread for children (and indeed many adults) that they may
  consider their pain to be preferable to the injections. *The IM route is
  therefore to be avoided in children*

- parenteral route (SC, IV). If the parenteral route is chosen, the mode of delivery must be considered:
  - *continuous infusions* avoid the problems of peaks and troughs associated with
  - *intermittent dosing*, which may lead to alternating periods of unacceptable side effects and breakthrough pain, especially if given on a p.r.n. basis
  - this problem may be overcome by *regular dosing* if equipment for infusions is not available, however the dosing interval must then be appropriate
  - consideration should be given to *patient controlled analgesia* (PCA) which gives patients the ability to control their pain to a steady state of their choosing. It must, however, be remembered that in some circumstances it is not always desirable to give full control to the patient; for instance a degree of sedation associated with opiate infusions might be warranted, especially in terminal disease[5]

- the intravenous route has the advantage of the rapidity with which analgesia can be titrated to control pain

- subcutaneous infusions and subcutaneous PCA have been used with good effect once pain is under control.[6] The equipment can be simple and portable and may be used as an alternative to intravenous infusions. Cannulae usually need changing every three to five days; the advent of topical local anaesthetic creams makes replacing the cannula much less stressful than it has been in the past

- neuraxial (spinal and/or epidural) administration is the most invasive route for drug delivery. This degree of invasiveness is unwarranted in most children but in a small proportion this route may have to be considered.

Indications for using neuraxial techniques are listed in Box 10.2.

Neuraxial techniques can be achieved with the use of indwelling, tunnelled catheters, and lightweight portable pumps to deliver a continuous infusion.[8] Both local anaesthetics and opiates have been used and some patients can be managed at home once the regimen is established.

The above section concentrates on analgesic pharmacology but these are not the only agents that are used to manage chronic pain. Chronic pain can both manifest itself and be responsible for depressive illness. In adults antidepressants are frequently used in the management of chronic pain but they are used much less in children. As well as their antidepressant actions some evidence exists that these agents have some intrinsic analgesic properties; if other analgesic regimens are not succeeding it may be worth considering the addition of an antidepressant to the treatment regimen. However, as with so

---

Box 10.2   Indications for neuraxial techniques[7]

- Poor pain control associated with excessive sedation, respiratory depression or disorientation in spite of high dose opiates and appropriate adjuncts

- All other non-invasive options (physiotherapy, psychotherapy) have proved unhelpful

- The presence of deafferentation pain unrelieved by drugs and TENS

- Incisional and visceral pain following surgery

- Prevention of phantom limb pain[2]

---

much in this field, there are very few paediatric trials on which to base choice scientifically.

Non-drug therapies

These therapies are only discussed briefly as a full discussion can be found in Chapter 7. These therapies should not be considered as alternatives to each other, or to the more paternalistic, 'traditional' medical approach, but rather all have a greater or lesser role to play in managing a child in pain. Non-drug methods should be used in conjunction with pharmacological methods.

Psychological therapy

There are several types of psychological approach to children. The technique chosen depends mainly on the experience and training of the therapist. The psychological therapies available for treating chronic pain in children can be seen in Box 10.3.

Physical therapy

The physical therapies available for treating chronic pain in children can be seen in Box 10.4.

Having given an overview of the options available for the management of chronic pain, these will be applied to practice by looking at several conditions that can result in chronic pain in children.

Box 10.3 Psychological therapies

Operant conditioning	• A technique to modify pain behaviours rather than be directed towards the pain *per se*
Cognitive-behavioural therapy	• Developed from the recognition that cognition and emotion play a central role in the experience of pain
	• An active process for the patient and entails the learning of cognitive and behavioural skills aimed at reducing negative emotions and thoughts associated with a painful experience and thus reducing the suffering and pain behaviour previously produced by pain
	• Psychologists will be able to identify and augment existing strategies and introduce new ones as they deem appropriate, as well as discourage negative strategies adopted by the child
	• Psychological techniques used would include distraction, relaxation and imagery (guided or otherwise)
	• This latter technique may be particularly suitable for younger children where the boundaries of reality and fantasy are often blurred
Biofeedback	• Requires the patient to learn how to influence a physiological response that has been detected and amplified into a form that is easily sensed
	• Mainly used for headaches
Hypnosis	

Sickle-cell disease

The pain associated with sickle-cell disease is highly variable.[9] Its duration can be hours to weeks and its severity mild to severe (even more so than post-operative pain). Indeed, some of the African tribal names for the disease express its painful nature, for example 'body chewing', 'body biting', 'beaten up'.

Box 10.4   Physical therapies

Physiotherapy	• In its purest sense physiotherapy is involved with maintaining or improving function, through exercise or passive movement of soft tissues, which has a role in several chronic, painful conditions such as chronic arthritis
	• Physiotherapists have also become involved with other physical therapies
Thermotherapy	• This is the application of heat by direct or indirect methods and the removal of heat, for example the application of cold packs
	• Indirect methods of heat application involve microwaves, ultrasound and warm baths
TENS	• Has its basis for use in the 'gate-control' theory of pain
	• By stimulating the A fibres (fast conducting) these inhibit presynaptically the slower conducting C fibres thus preventing or reducing passage of pain messages to the central nervous system
	• This is achieved by delivering a current (usually 50 mA) at a frequency (usually 80–100 Hz) for a time (0.05–0.2 milliseconds)
	• The exact settings and position of the electrodes can be determined with the child. Its use, in adults, is widespread more due to its lack of severe side effects rather than clinically based trials but some patients do gain benefit from its use

---

It may be argued that the inclusion of sickle-cell disease (SCD) in a chapter about chronic pain is inappropriate as SCD is characterized by intermittent acutely painful episodes which should be treated as such. Whilst this is undoubtedly true and the management of the pain follows an acute model, the chronicity of the condition, and the associated psychological problems, lends itself to consideration in this chapter.

Pathophysiology

• SCD occurs as a result of an inherited alteration in the genetic code for the b globin subunit of the haemoglobin molecule.

- There are several different sickling haemoglobinopathies depending on the exact alteration of the amino acid sequence, which may in part explain the variation in severity of crises between individuals.

- The condition affects about 1 in 600 of the population whose ancestors come from areas where malaria is endemic, in particular the African and Indian continents and areas of the Mediterranean basin.

- The protection of fetal haemoglobin disappears by the age of six to nine months. Subsequently, painful episodes may begin; pain is the commonest presenting problem in children.[10]

- In children under three this is usually pain in the fingers and toes and in adolescents there is abdominal pain.

- The pain is caused by vaso-occlusive crises resulting in an acute episode of pain followed by a return to the child's baseline pain state.

Clinical course

- Some are fortunate and have only occasional painful episodes, which may be approached along the lines of any acute pain episode as described in Chapter 8.

- Others have frequent and/or severe pain, which intrudes into the everyday life of themselves and their families. This is a chronic pain syndrome as it is likely to be lifelong.

- In such cases the management of the sufferer requires the integration of:
  - pharmacological
  - psychological
  - behavioural
  - physical approaches.

This needs to involve both the patient and his or her family.

Any disease that causes repetitive, unavoidable and unpredictable episodes of pain may lead to a perception of lack of control over life events leading to a 'learned helplessness'.[11] When this happens during childhood and adolescence it may alter a child's concept of independence and body image and there is evidence of significant psychopathology and social dysfunction in patients with sickle-cell disease.[12] Thus early intervention is necessary to try to minimize problems later in life.

Assessment

- There is no reliable marker to distinguish vaso-occlusive pain from any other pain.

- The pain assessment tools described in Chapters 5 and 6 must be used.

- The practitioner must never fail to consider the possibility that the child's pain is not 'crisis pain'; older children are themselves able to distinguish a different quality to the pain of their crises.

- Once an assessment has been made, pain relief should be instituted.

Treatment

Although control of the pain itself is of the utmost importance from a symptomatic and humanitarian standpoint, there are other important facets of treatment:

- diagnosis and treatment of cause

- appropriate control of fluid balance

- the role of oxygen.

Pharmacological therapy

The approach to treating the painful crisis depends on how severe the pain is, what background level of pain the child has and the regular treatment that the child is taking. These factors themselves may be modified depending on the child's family support, social and ethnic background.

- As pain management is unlikely to be instituted by an anaesthetist in this situation, it is of benefit for protocols to be available to which other health care professionals may refer in order that appropriate analgesia is given (Figure 10.1).

- The two arms in Figure 10.1 are not to be treated as exclusive alternatives, as combinations of agents (opioids, simple analgesics and adjuvants) may prove more beneficial than a single agent alone. It must be borne in mind that this is only one example of a protocol for the management of the acute stage of the painful episode.

- Oral opioids are available and it may be appropriate to use these to stage withdrawal from intravenous opioids, which may allow the child home earlier.

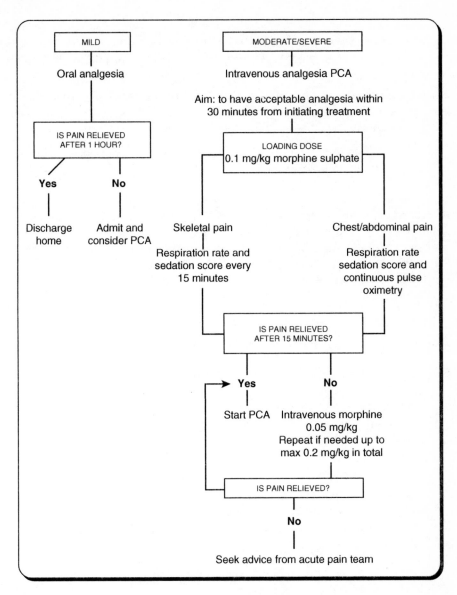

Figure 10.1:   Example of a pain protocol for children with sickle-cell disease.

- Some concern has been voiced about the potential for opioid-induced respiratory depression and hypoxia to prolong a crisis. However, the co-administration of oxygen and the advent of patient controlled analgesia (PCA) technology make this less likely to be a major problem.

- The doses of morphine used may be high and, if PCA is used, frequent re-evaluation is needed to optimize bolus doses and lockout times. This is where the skill of a dedicated acute pain team may be of value.

- Using PCA in this situation has the added psychological benefit of giving control of the pain to the child.

There is one case report of epidural analgesia being used but its frequent use is not indicated unless the painful episode is particularly severe or side effects from other agents are a major problem.[13] It is not known how often epidural catheters can be sited and the technique may be distressing for smaller children. Use of this technique may also undermine some of the non-drug approaches that can be used for pain management (see below).

Non-drug methods of pain relief

- *Cognitive-behavioural therapy and psychological methods.* There is potential for significant psychopathology in patients with sickle-cell disease and psychological help should be introduced early. This needs to be appropriate for the child's age and needs (meditation will not work for a one year-old) and must be compatible with the child's own coping strategy. If it is left too late before using these approaches, learned behaviour develops making them more difficult to use.

- *Hypnosis and biofeedback* have been used frequently and, whilst no con-trolled trials have been performed, they are relatively easy to learn and are free of side effects.[14]

- *Warm packs and baths* may be beneficial.

- *TENS* has been used although it has not been shown to decrease the length of time spent in hospital.[15]

- *Education of the family* about the disease itself and about pain man-agement strategies is as important as the management itself and allows treatment to be tailored to the individual.

It may be useful to draw up a contract between patients and their families and health care professionals in which dose and schedule of medication, self-care criteria, admission criteria and weaning are all formalized. Although this may appear excessively formal, such contracts have been seen to be of benefit particularly to adolescents.[16]

Follow up

Once over the acute episode, the patient and family need to be counselled and supported in order that disrupted social activity and lost time at school are caught up to prevent the cycle of underachievement and social dysfunction that may often ensue.

Cancer pain and terminal care

The pattern of cancer pain in paediatrics is different from that found in adult cancer.

- Sixty to 70 per cent of adults with cancer have pain directly related to their cancers; in children direct pain occurs in only about 25% of cases.[17]

- Painful episodes are more likely to be due to therapy and procedures (50%).

- A significant amount of pain (25% of cases) is completely unrelated to the cancer.[18]

The reasons suggested for this difference are:

- the different spectrum of malignancies in children

- the rapidity of tumour regression once treatment is commenced

- the relatively long duration of disease-free survival, making procedure-related pain proportionately more memorable

- the rapidity with which children succumb to non-responding malignancies.[7]

Having made an assessment of the child, treatment should commence without delay with the aim of obtaining rapid pain control by whatever means are appropriate. Only once treatment of pain has been initiated should further investigations be carried out.

> The degree of investigation must be appropriate to the situation. It may be inappropriate to investigate thoroughly a child who is entering the terminal phase of his illness. On the other hand, detailed investigation may be appropriate if it is possible that the cause of the pain is treatable, as this may improve the quality of the last few weeks of life.

In the light of the results of the investigations a definitive plan can be formulated. The nature of the plan will depend on the cause of the pain. The pain will be:

- cancer-related – for example, bone pain, nerve pain, visceral pain
- therapy-related – for example, nerve pain, phantom pain, mucositis
- unrelated to the malignancy.

The treatment of cancer-related pain is primarily directed at the malignancy itself. Thus the patient should undergo chemotherapy, radiotherapy or surgery as appropriate under the supervision of the oncologists.

If the pain is related to therapy or apparently unrelated to the malignancy it may have an obvious cause, in which case the treatment is directed at this. The pain may, however, have no obvious cause in which case treatment is aimed at alleviating pain empirically along the lines outlined at the beginning of the chapter.

Musculoskeletal pain

> By definition this is pain related to bones, joints, muscles and connective tissue.
>
> It is estimated that approximately 15% of children will suffer musculo-skeletal pain at some stage in their childhood.
>
> The causes of musculoskeletal pain are legion and cover a large breadth of paediatric sub-disciplines.

The great difficulty for health care professionals is to sift those cases of severe or life-threatening illness from the rest. As with so many areas of medical practice this relies on:

- a detailed history of the pain itself
- a family history, in case of genetic predisposition

- a social history, which may help to reveal the possible existence of pain with no physical cause.

In addition, a careful examination is mandatory to assess the part played in the aetiology of the pain by:

- nerves
- the vasculature
- bones and joints.

Juvenile rheumatoid arthritis

This condition affects nine to 14 per 100 000 children and usually first occurs between one to three years of age. The underlying pathology is one of chronic synovial inflammation.

The presenting symptoms and signs depend, like so much in paediatrics, on:

- the age and cognitive development of the child
- the severity of the pain
- social factors
- the emotional state of the child.

The main symptoms are:

- stiffness and pain particularly after inactivity
- a limp or, in the younger child, refusal to crawl or walk at all.

The child may also exhibit other non-specific features that may exacerbate the misery they feel due to the pain:

- fever
- rashes
- swollen lymph nodes
- anaemia.

Several sub-types of juvenile arthritis have been reported depending on:

- the chronicity of the disease
- the pain
- the severity of joint involvement
- the degree of systemic upset.

It is, however, pain that is the consistent predictor of the physical and psychological outcome; the pain therefore needs adequate assessment and treatment.[19]

Pain in children with juvenile rheumatoid arthritis may be assessed using the Varni–Thompson Pain Questionnaire.[20] It should be remembered that it is not only the current pain that needs to be addressed but other factors that have an effect on the severity of pain perception:

- functional status of the child
- family variables
- psychological adjustment of the child.

Addressing problems within these areas may allow for an improvement in long-term pain control with lower doses of pharmacological agents.

The pain associated with juvenile arthritis can be:

- related to the disease process itself
- secondary to treatment, for example physiotherapy
- unrelated to the disease.

There are two major modalities of treatment: pharmacological methods and non-drug methods.

Pharmacological methods

These are undoubtedly the mainstay of treatment and are widely accepted to include:

- aspirin or other anti-inflammatory drugs, which are thought to work by reducing the production of prostaglandins that sensitize nerve endings resulting in pain from otherwise trivial stimuli

- these are successful in treating the inflammatory process adequately in 60–75% of children

- the remainder may go on to receive second-line, disease-modifying agents such as penicillamine, gold and hydroxychloroquine.

Non-drug methods

There are two major approaches:

- physiotherapy. The rationale is to limit contracture formation and aim at the long-term adaptation of the child to his or her condition. The treatment itself can cause significant pain and it is difficult for younger children to separate the two. Thus the child gets pain with physiotherapy and pain is perceived as bad and so physiotherapy must be bad. It is here that one has to involve the family in order that the treatment continues and to use the second of the non-drug approaches

- cognitive-behavioural therapy. This is discussed in Chapter 7.

Neuropathic pain

Neuropathic pain in children usually follows an injury of some description (which may have been relatively trivial). This leaves the child with a degree of impaired function, usually of a limb, and with areas of skin that have altered sensation. This may be altered in quality or sensitivity. The pain is usually described in terms of burning, pins and needles or tingling, and is often pain caused by a stimulus that is not usually pain-provoking (allodynia).

It is important to make a proper evaluation in order to rule out treatable causes of neuropathies, but these are not common in children. The advice of a neurologist can be invaluable. Treatment can be very difficult, may be prolonged and may involve a certain amount of trial and error in order to improve the pain. Indeed palliation and rehabilitation may have to be the goal.

The two major examples of non-cancer-related neuropathic pain in children are:

- reflex sympathetic dystrophy

- amputation pain.

Reflex sympathetic dystrophy is:

- a burning type of pain
- associated with autonomic dysfunction
- associated with trophic changes.

Clinical features

- It usually follows injury, which may have been trivial.
- It is more common in girls.
- It is rarely seen under nine years of age.
- It affects lower limbs more often than upper ones.

Assessment and treatment

- Thermography has been used to delineate the autonomic dysfunction but is only a diagnostic tool.
- Sympathetic blockade, in contrast, is both diagnostic and therapeutic. Intravenous phentolamine (an a-adrenoceptor blocker) has been used as a diagnostic tool prior to undertaking a therapeutic sympathetic blockade.
- The above allow active and pain-free physiotherapy, which maintains the limb in good functional order.
- Physiotherapy should be combined with psychological and cognitive-behavioural therapy, for both the individual and his or her family, with the aim of reversing the 'disability syndrome' that often accompanies this condition.

In contrast to the case in adults, reflex sympathetic dystrophy usually improves over time.

Amputation pain

In the context of chronic pain, this is not the post-operative pain of any surgical procedure but comprises stump pain and phantom limb pain. A painful stump may have an underlying cause such as a neuroma or an infection that needs treating along surgical lines. Phantom limb sensations may be more prevalent in children than adults and it is important to remember that not all phantom sensation is necessarily painful.[23] Pre-emptive treatment has been suggested to reduce the incidence of phantom limb pain in adults but the causes of adult amputation present a different spectrum of disease and so the results may be different.[24]

Treatment

Treatment methods are myriad for phantom limb pain, which suggests the poor efficacy of any of them. They can be classified as follows:

- pharmacological – standard analgesics both opiate and non-opiate, and other adjuvant drugs (anticonvulsants, antidepressants). Tricyclic anti-depressants have been used in adults, as have antiepileptics such as carbamazepine. Children may be suffering a different kind of pain and only a few studies have used these drugs for neuropathic pain in children. The notable thing about neuropathic pain is that it may be resistant to opioids[22]
- regional blocks – diagnostic and therapeutic
- physical therapies – TENS, heat, acupuncture
- psychological
- surgery – this should only be considered for a specific surgically treatable cause of the pain as it has no objective benefit over any of the other modalities.

It has to be noted that the necessary controlled clinical trials have not been carried out and so, ultimately, treatment is based on trial and error and a doctor's past experience of dealing with this condition and it may not be successful.

Headaches

Headaches are the commonest of all chronic pain syndromes.

A survey carried out in 1962 showed that up to 75% of children will complain of headache at some time.[25]

The challenge in this situation is to separate those headaches with organic causes from those with no organic cause. In children this is always difficult since some children with no organic cause for their headaches may subsequently develop an organic headache. Fortunately this is usually heralded by a change in the nature and severity of the headache and the development of other signs and symptoms.

A good history and detailed examination must be carried out whilst paying attention to other clues such as the effect on the child and family and the interaction between them. Any neurological abnormality needs full investigation as a matter of urgency; this usually involves a CT or MRI scan. Other investigations depend on the likely differential diagnosis. Headaches that are acute, recurrent and/or progressively more severe and headaches that occur early in the morning are more likely to be associated with pathology than chronic non-progressive headaches.

Treatment is primarily directed at any underlying cause. This leaves a group of children with chronic non-progressive headaches with no neurological symptoms and signs and negative investigations and it includes a preponderance of adolescent females. This group needs an open discussion of the non-pathological nature of the headache and a social and psychological appraisal of the family can often be of benefit. Psychological modes of treatment often in conjunction with psychiatric treatment for depression (which may be primary or secondary to the headache) are frequently most productive.[26]

Multi-disciplinary approach

It is well recognized that a multi-disciplinary approach to the management of chronic pain in adults works well. This is because:

- it employs the expertise of several specialists allowing a broad base for diagnostic evaluation and an integrated approach to pain management (psychological, medical, physiotherapy and 'alternative' therapies)

- it has the advantage of avoiding the slow process of multiple referrals and repeated investigations

- there is nothing to suggest that this approach is any less appropriate for children

- nurses have a central role in that they have closer and more prolonged contact with the patient and family than any other health care professional

- much of the information to be gleaned about a child in pain comes from the nurses caring for the child

- it includes the scoring of pain but also the behavioural responses of the child and family to the pain, and to each other, and to treatment itself

- the close involvement of nurses allows an objective assessment of any ongoing treatment.

This multi-disciplinary approach has two other advantages:

- it allows the family to be involved at an early stage in dealing and coping with a child with chronic pain
- it brings together health care professionals with an interest in pain, allowing a greater exchange of ideas and provoking further research into the causes and treatment of chronic painful conditions in childhood.

Summary

- The management of chronic pain in children can be more difficult than in adults for a number of reasons.
- Chronic pain is pain which persists beyond the usual course of an acute disease or which is associated with an underlying chronic condition.
- When considering how to treat pain it is important to try to ascertain the cause of the pain.
- Pain control can be provided by pharmacological and non-drug methods.
- There are a number of routes by which analgesic drugs can be administered; consideration needs to be given to the most appropriate.
- Non-drug methods should be used in conjunction with the pharmacological methods.
- A multi-disciplinary approach needs to be adopted.

References

1   Melzack R (1990) The tragedy of needless pain. *Sci Am.* **262**: (2) 27–33.
2   Bonica JJ (1953) *The Management of Pain.* Lea & Febiger, Pennsylvania.
3   WHO (1990) *Cancer pain relief and palliative care.* WHO Technical Report Series 804. WHO, Geneva.
4   Miser AW, Narong PK, Dothage JA *et al.* (1989) Transdermal fentanyl for pain control in patients with cancer. *Pain.* **37**: 15–21.
5   Miser AW *et al.* (1980) Continuous infusions of morphine sulphate for control of severe pain in children with terminal malignancy. *J Paediatr.* **96**: 930–2.
6   Miser AW *et al.* (1983) Continuous subcutaneous infusions of morphine in children with cancer. *Am J Dis Child.* **137**: 383–5.

7   Miser AW (1993) Management of pain associated with childhood cancer. In: *Pain in Infants, Children and Adolescents* (eds NL Schechter, CB Berde and M Yaster). Williams & Wilkins, Baltimore.

8   Berde CB (1989) Regional analgesia in the management of chronic pain in childhood. *J Pain Symptom Manage.* **4**: 232–7.

9   Shapiro B, Dinges DF and Orne ED (1990) Recording of crisis pain in sickle cell disease. In: *Advances in Pain Research and Therapy* (eds D Tyler and E Krane). Raven Press, New York.

10   Brozavic M, Davies S and Brownell A (1987) Acute admissions of patients with sickle cell disease who live in Britain. *BMJ.* **294**: 1206–8.

11   Maier SF and Seligman MEP (1976) Learned helplessness: theory and evidence. *J Exp Psychol.* **105**: 3–46.

12   Damlouji NF, Georgopoulos A, Kevess-Cohen R *et al.* (1982) Social disability and psychiatric morbidity in sickle cell anaemia and diabetes patients. *Psychosomatics.* **23**: 925–31.

13   Finer P, Blain J and Rowe P (1988) Epidural analgesia in the management of labour pain and sickle cell crisis. *Anaesth.* **68**: 799–800.

14   Zeltzer L, Dash J and Holland JP (1979) Hypnotically induced pain control in sickle cell anaemia. *Paediatrics.* **12**: 51–61.

15   Wong WC, Parker LJ and George SL (1985) TENS treatment of sickle cell painful crises. *Blood.* **66** (suppl): 67a.

16   Burghardt-Fitzgerald DC (1989) Pain behaviour contracts: effective management of the adolescent in sickle cell crisis. *J Pediatr Nurs.* **4**: 320–4.

17   Daut RL and Cleeland CS (1982) The prevalence and severity of pain in cancer. *Cancer.* **50**: 1913–18.

18   Miser AW *et al.* (1987) The prevalence of pain in paediatric and young adult cancer populations. *Pain.* **29**: 73–83.

19   Lovell DJ and Walco GA (1989) Pain associated with juvenile rheumatoid arthritis. *Pediatr Clin North Am.* **36**: 1015–27.

20   Varni JW, Thompson KL and Hanson V (1987) The Varni-Thompson Pediatric Pain Questionnaire 1: chronic musculoskeletal pain in juvenile rheumatoid arthritis. *Pain.* **28**: 27–38.

21   Rogers AG (1984) Use of amitryptiline for phantom limb pain in younger children. *J Pain Symptom Manage.* **4**: 96.

22   Arner S and Meyerson BA (1989) Lack of analgesic effect of opioids on neuropathic and idiopathic forms of pain. *Pain.* **33**: 11–23.

23   Krane EJ, Heller LB and Pomietto ML (1991) Incidence of phantom sensation in paediatric amputees. *Anaesth.* **75**: A69.

24   Bach S, Noreg MF and Tjellden NV (1988) Phantom limb pain in amputees during the first 12 months following amputation and preoperative lumbar epidural blockade. *Pain.* **33**: 297–301.

25   Bille BS (1962) Migraine in school children. *Paediatrics.* **51** (suppl 136): 1–51.

26   Rothner AD (1978) Headaches in children. A review. *Headache.* **18** (3): 169.

11   The future of paediatric pain management

The best possible management of children's pain is a moral and ethical obligation for care givers; untreated pain has undesirable consequences,[1] yet as we approach the twenty-first century children are still suffering unnecessary pain during hospitalization.

Health care professionals should use their theoretical knowledge about paediatric pain management in their clinical practice to ensure that children no longer endure unnecessary pain. This chapter will first discuss ways of changing practice and then examine new advances in paediatric pain management. Areas where research is still required will also be identified and the management of change will be discussed.

Changing practice

The management of children's pain needs to become more aggressive. Changes are needed in hospital policy; education alone is not enough.[1]

Cummings *et al.*'s recommendations for improving the management of paediatric pain can be seen in Box 11.1.

There are several relatively simple ways of improving the management of paediatric pain which are identified in Box 11.2.

Those individuals who demonstrate the greatest insight regarding pain management for children are nurses with masters degrees. These nurses, however, because of managerial responsibilities, are often not closely involved in the actual delivery of care. In contrast, those nurses providing the most nursing care (that is those with the least nursing education) were found to hold the most misconceptions about effective pain management for children.[2]

Box 11.1   The recommendations of Cummings *et al.* (1996)[1]

- Children who are in the post-operative period, who have intravenous lines, who may have disease-related pain, or who have acute illness are easily identified and should be specifically targeted for intervention

- Sources of pain are often unique to the individual and difficult to predict

- Assessment and treatment of pain must be conducted on an individual basis

- Pain assessment should be approached with the same attention as that of vital signs

- The administration practices and effectiveness of medications must be assessed and monitored for each child (e.g. inclusion of a pain flow sheet in the hospital record)

- A change in physician pain management practices is necessary

- Education of all medical and nursing staff is a first step toward achievement of improved use of medication

- Hospital staff need educating in the use of psychological and non-drug techniques of pain control

- Parents should be educated and have resources available to them in hospital to assist them in assessing and managing their children's pain

- Significant improvement in the management of paediatric pain is unlikely to occur solely through attempts to educate individual health care professionals and parents

- Changes in hospital policy and practice are necessary; for example, education for all hospital staff combined with quality assurance procedures requiring documentation of pain assessment and treatment and ongoing audits

---

Box 11.2   Simple steps that can improve the management of paediatric pain

- Using a pain assessment tool

- Asking children how much pain they have

- Observing the child's non-verbal behavioural clues

- Encouraging parents to be involved

- Writing an information leaflet for parents

- Minimizing the use of intra-muscular injections

- Having a range of analgesic drugs available

- Using non-drug methods of pain control

- Writing a standard of care for pain management

- Auditing the standard

There is a need for better and continuing education about paediatric pain for all health care professionals. There is a need for the amount of content about paediatric pain in curricula to be re-evaluated; one reason why pain management is not seen as a priority by health care professionals is perhaps the lack of input they received in pre-registration training. There is also a need for a greater number of post-registration courses about paediatric pain.

Misconceptions about paediatric pain are still prevalent in clinical practice today.[1-5]

As well as improving education there are several steps that need to be taken in order to challenge health care professionals' misconceptions regarding paediatric pain.[1-5] The steps that need to be taken can be seen in Box 11.3.

Education alone is not sufficient to change people's behaviour about a phenomenon. An increase in theoretical knowledge about pain management does not necessarily lead to changes in clinical practices.[7]

Box 11.3   Steps that need to be taken to address misconceptions about paediatric pain[1-5]

- Provision of education for nurses in clinical practice in a formal setting – i.e. away from the clinical area

- A clinical protocol (or pain resource manual) needs to be written

- A team approach needs to be taken by the multi-disciplinary team – i.e. the involvement of anaesthetists and nursing staff at all levels within the organization

- A clinical nurse specialist in paediatric pain to facilitate the education of nurses and other health care professionals, the writing of protocols, and to support and challenge the nurses in the clinical areas

- Availability of an anaesthetist – daily ward round and on a bleep

---

(These recommendations are supported by the US DHHS (1992) guidelines for Acute Pain Management in Infants, Children and Adolescents.)[6]

- Changing beliefs and attitudes is never easy.

- This perhaps explains why in spite of compelling evidence health care professionals continue to believe the misconceptions about paediatric pain.

- Attitudes are relatively stable entities but are not fixed. They change and can be changed.[8]

Ways need to be found to change attitudes about paediatric pain; education alone is not enough. It is also necessary to find methods of changing behaviour and for facilitating evidence-based practice.

Advances in paediatric pain management

Pharmacological advances

A number of new drugs have been developed or are in the process of being developed.

Propacetamol

This is an injectable form of paracetamol that has been used successfully in France and Belgium for a number of years and will hopefully be introduced into the UK soon.[9] The recommended dose is 30 mg/kg of intravenous propacetamol administered over 15 minutes, given every 6 hours. There are no significant differences in pharmacokinetics in children or adults. The clearance is prolonged in neonates.[10]

The advantages of propacetamol in children are:

• it may be used when the gastrointestinal system is not functioning

• it has a shorter onset time

• it is more effective than oral paracetamol.[9]

Tramadol

• Used extensively in continental Europe.

• An agonist at opiate receptors that produces less respiratory depression than opiates in comparable doses.[11]

• At present unlicensed for use in children below the age of 12 years.

• Anecdotal evidence suggests that it produces a high incidence of nausea and vomiting, which may decrease its usefulness.

Ketamine

An established drug that has been used safely for anaesthesia. Recently the use of ketamine in addition to caudal bupivacaine has been demonstrated.[12] Ketamine has been found to be an effective analgesic drug.

• The children who had ketamine added to caudal bupivacaine had significantly more sleep on their first night after minor surgery than those who just had bupivacaine.[12]

• The ketamine available in the UK, at the moment, is mixed with a preservative (benzethonium chloride).

• There is work to suggest that the combination of ketamine and preservative is neurotoxic.

• The preservative in this instance was chlorbutanol, which is used in the USA, rather than benzethonium chloride.[13]

- This may still prevent the use of ketamine as an additive but it is hoped that a form of ketamine will be produced which can be added to caudal bupivacaine safely.

Ropivacaine

An amide-type local anaesthetic that has a number of advantages over bupivacaine:

- it is less toxic, which means that higher concentrations can be used[14]

- when higher concentrations (1%) of ropivacaine are used the nerve block is more effective and lasts longer than 0.5% bupivacaine[15]

- it has less effect on sensory nerves than bupivacaine, resulting in better mobility with epidural infusions[16]

- it may be used as the sole agent for epidural infusion analgesia, reducing the incidence of itching, nausea and urinary retention.

Anecdotally, the use of ropivacaine as a sole agent in epidural infusions produces its own problems:

- the catheter needs to be sited at the level of vertebra corresponding to the pain dermatome. For example, the catheter tip needs to be at approximately T10/11 for use in abdominal surgery

- to produce complete analgesia a NSAID needs to be given in conjunction with the infusion of ropivacaine.

Many of the drugs that are used in the care of children are administered by a route, in a formulation or in a dosage that has not been approved by the Medicines Control Agency. Steps need to be taken to rectify this situation; drugs used in the treatment of children need to be licensed.

Royal College of Paediatrics and Child Health guidelines

The Royal College of Paediatrics and Child Health (formerly the British Paediatric Association) have recently published guidelines for the management of pain in children.[17] The book discusses both physiological and psychological aspects of pain management as well as providing advice on the administration of analgesic drugs. It is hoped that the book will enable health care professionals to manage pain in children more effectively.

The Children's Charter

'You can expect to be told what pain relief will be given to your child to make his or her stay in hospital as comfortable as possible.'[18]

While it is encouraging that parents' need for information is addressed within *The Children's Charter* this does not appear to address issues pertinent to pain management or require much commitment on the part of health care professionals. It is hoped that these issues will be addressed in the future revisions of the Charter.[18]

Areas for further research

There are several areas where further research is required. These include:

- the priority given to pain management by health care professionals
- the educational content of pre-registration courses
- children's understanding and perception of their pain
- management of specific types of pain,* for example:
  - trauma pain
  - sickle-cell pain
  - rheumatoid arthritis pain
- the effectiveness of non-drug pain control methods
- ways of changing the perceptions and behaviour of health care professionals.

Management of change

George Bernard Shaw stated that all progress depends on the *unreasonable* person. Reasonable people adapt themselves to the world while unreasonable people persist in trying to adapt the world to themselves; therefore, for any change of consequence we must look to the unreasonable person.[19]

* Much has been written about the management of post-operative pain and the management of cancer pain in children has in the past few years been researched more thoroughly, however there is a need to highlight the management of other types of pain.

In implementing a strategy to improve pain management it is important to remember that change is involved:

- change is always difficult

- change is always a challenge and there is invariably resistance

- this resistance is usually due to fear and misinformation[20]

- maintaining clear communication channels in wards and organizations can therefore be seen to be important in managing change.

This book has provided the information required to facilitate the required changes in practice. For practice to change, however, commitment to change is needed from both those working in the clinical area and from their managers. It is only when behaviours as well as beliefs are altered that children will no longer endure unnecessary pain.[21]

It will not be easy but health care professionals must work together to ensure that the required changes in perceptions and practices do happen; it is no longer acceptable for children to be enduring unnecessary pain.

> The challenge for paediatric health care providers in the late 1990s is not only to be informed of current practices in pain and symptom control, but also to remember to establish those practices in day-to-day management.[21]

Summary

- Children are still suffering unnecessary pain.

- Health care professionals have a moral obligation to provide the best possible management of children's pain.

- There are several relatively simple ways of improving the management of paediatric pain.

- Better education is needed at the pre- and post-registration level.

- Health care professionals' misconceptions about paediatric pain need to be challenged.

- Behaviours need to change.

- There are a number of pharmacological advances that although in need of further evaluation will, it is hoped, further improve the management of pain in children.

- The guidelines recently published by the Royal College of Paediatrics and Child Health are an important step in ensuring that children no longer endure unnecessary pain.

- While parents' need for information is identified in *The Children's Charter* it is hoped that future editions will go further.

- There is still a need for research into many areas of paediatric pain management.

- In effecting change it is necessary to consider how this change is managed.

References

1   Cummings EA, Reid GJ, Finley A *et al.* (1996) Prevalence and source of pain in pediatric inpatients. *Pain.* **68**: 25–31.

2   Margolius FR, Hudson KA and Michel Y (1995) Beliefs and perceptions about children in pain: a survey. *Pediatr Nurs.* **21** (2): 111–15.

3   Schmidt K, Eland J and Weller K (1994) Pediatric cancer pain management: a survey of nurses' knowledge. *J Pediatr Oncol.* **11** (1): 4–12.

4   Woodgate R and Kristjanson LJ (1996) A young child's pain: how parents and nurses 'take care'. *Int J Nurs Stud.* **33** (3): 271–84.

5   Twycross A (1995) Children's nursing in Canada. *Paediatr Nurs.* **7** (4): 8–10, May.

6   US DHHS (1992) *Acute Pain Management in Infants, Children and Adolescents: Operative and Medical Procedures.* DHSS.

7   McGrath PJ (1996) Attitudes and beliefs about medication and pain management in children. *J Palliat Care.* **12** (3): 46–50.

8   Downie RS, Fyfe C and Tannahill A (1990) *Health Promotion: Models and Values.* Oxford Medical Publications, Oxford.

9   Boccard E, Jardé O, Hayek J *et al.* (1993) Compared analgesic efficacy of an injectable prodrug of acetaminophen with oral acetaminophen after hallux valgus plasty. Seventh World Congress on Pain, August 22–27. Book of abstracts, **61**: Abstract 171.

10   Murat I, Granry J and Camboulives J (1997) Therapeutic use of propacetamol hydrochloride. In: *Proceedings of the symposium on propacetamol*, 4th European Congress of Paediatric Anaesthesia, pp. 39–48.

11   Bösenberg AT and Ratcliffe S (1997) Respiratory effects of tramadol in children under halothane anaesthesia. In: *Book of Abstracts of the 4th European Congress of Paediatric Anaesthesia.* p. 38.

12   Cook B, Grubb DJ, Aldridge LA *et al.* (1995) Comparison of the effects of adrenaline, clonidine and ketamine on the duration of caudal analgesia produced by bupivacaine in children. *Br J Anaesth.* **75** (6): 698–701.

13   Malinovsky J, Cozian A, Lepage J *et al.* (1991) Ketamine and midazolam neuro-toxicity in the rabbit. *Anesthesiology.* **75**: 91–7.
14   Scott DB, Lee A, Fagan, D *et al.* (1989) Acute toxicity of ropivacaine compared with that of bupivacaine. *Anesth Analg.* **69**: 563–9.
15   Wolff AP, Hasselström L, Kerkkamp HE *et al.* (1995) Extradural ropivacaine and bupivacaine in hip surgery. *Br J Anaesth.* **74**: 458–60.
16   Schug SA, Scott DA, Payne J *et al.* (1996) Postoperative analgesia by continuous extradural infusion of ropivacaine after upper abdominal surgery. *Br J Anaesth.* **76**: 487–91.
17   Royal College of Paediatrics and Child Health (1997) *Prevention and Control of Pain in Children.* BMJ Publishing Group, London.
18   Department of Health (1996) *Services for Children and Young People.* HMSO, London.
19   Shaw GB (1989) In: *The Age of Unreason* (ed. C Handy). Arrow Books, London.
20   Lancaster J and Lancaster W (eds) (1982) *The nurse as a change agent.* CV Mosby, St Louis.
21   Stevens MM, Pozza LD, Cavalletto B *et al.* (1994) Pain and symptom control in paediatric palliative care. In: *Cancer Surveys Volume 21: Palliative Medicine: Problem Areas in Pain and Symptom Management* (ed. GW Hanks). Cold Spring Harbor Laboratory Press.

Index

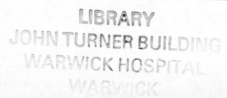